CURCUMIN

NATURE'S ANSWER TO

CANCER AND OTHER CHRONIC DISEASES

AJAY GOEL, PH.D.

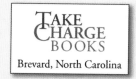

TAKE
CHARGE
BOOKS

Brevard, North Carolina

The purpose of this book is to educate. It is not intended to serve as a replacement for professional medical advice. Any use of the information in this book is at the reader's discretion. This book is sold with the understanding that neither the publisher nor the author has any liability or responsibility for any injury caused or alleged to be caused directly or indirectly by the information contained in this book. While every effort has been made to ensure its accuracy, the book's contents should not be construed as medical advice. To obtain medical advice on your individual health needs, please consult a qualified health care practitioner.

Library of Congress Cataloging-in Publication Data is on file with the Library of Congress.

ISBN: 978-0-9961589-1-6

Cover & interior: Gary A. Rosenberg • www.thebookcouple.com
Editor: Kathleen Barnes • www.takechargebooks.com

Printed in the United States of America

10   9   8   7   6   5   4   3   2   1

This book is dedicated to my family: my wife Shivali and my sons Akul and Arul, with love and gratitude for your patience, support and encouragement throughout all the years.

Contents

Acknowledgments

I sincerely and deeply appreciate each one of my mentors, colleagues, collaborators, research fellows and friends for teaching me and being there for me over the years. My research has truly been a team effort. I am indebted to each one of them for their valued contributions.

Jacob Teitelbaum, M.D.

Standard medicine has its strengths in treating acute medical emergencies such as appendicitis, heart attacks, antibiotic sensitive infections (e.g., pneumonias) and severe traumatic injuries. In these areas, it can truly shine and be lifesaving. Unfortunately, when it comes to treating chronic illness, including many cancers, standard medicine is often inadequately effective, and other branches of the healing arts may have much more to offer. Overall people have the most optimal outcomes when they combine the best of all branches of the healing arts.

In fact, the list of problems for which effective treatment is lacking is shrinking rapidly for just this reason.

A Turning Point

A major frustration for me when reading research on natural remedies was that curcumin (the active component of turmeric, the spice that makes Indian curry yellow) is one of the most powerful herbs for a wide variety of chronic diseases, including cancer.

The discovery of a method of making curcumin easily absorbed by the human body, a formulation called BCM-95™ has revolutionized medicine. It is the only formulation I will use because one pill can replace 14 of the next best curcumin formulation and an astounding 700 turmeric pills.

My friend and colleague, Dr. Ajay Goel, a noted cancer researcher at Baylor University, has written what I consider the most comprehensive book to date detailing the preventive and curative effects of curcumin against cancer and other chronic disease.

The Curcumin Cure

Let's look at a few examples of where the herb curcumin shows tremendous promise:

Chronic pain and fatigue. Having treated thousands of people with severe chronic pain, I can count on my fingers the ones for whom I've not been able to get adequate relief. This is also the experience of many pain specialists who combine a wide range of modalities. Many doctors turn to a variety of over-the-counter and prescription drugs with a variety of serious side effects that cause over 40,000 unnecessary deaths a year. Instead of side effects and tens of thousands of preventable deaths, we get ZERO deaths and instead of negative side effects, we get "side benefits" with curcumin.

Alzheimer's disease and dementia. The usually recommended prescription medications do not generally improve function. Instead, they slightly slow down progression. Yet the effectiveness of curcumin for improving function is astounding. Consider this: The prevalence of Alzheimer's is 70% lower in India due to the daily consumption of curcumin in the Indian diet.

And then of course, there is cancer. Though some standard chemo and radiation therapy regimens can be lifesaving, most are not curative. Sadly, some may do more harm than good, given with the attitude "Well, we have to do SOMETHING!"

The good news? People do best when their cancer is addressed with a number of synergistic treatments in combination. Dr. Goel's research confirms this. His results and those of a host of other researchers confirm that curcumin attacks cancer from several directions at once, making it unique in the arsenal against cancer.

We have problematic quirks in our health regulatory system that require safe and natural herbals to go through the same $400+ million regulatory process as drugs, making it essentially impossible for low cost natural products to do so. These quirks will eventually be fixed—but not in time for most people with cancer.

Fortunately, people don't have to wait, and can find the life saving research they need now with the simple "bottom line" information Dr. Goel offers right here in this book.

Thousands of studies and reports are finding that highly absorbed curcumin shows incredible promise for a wide array of cancers – both for prevention and treatment. In many, the effect is far greater than that of chemo and radiation and is synergistic with the standard medical therapies with no negative side effects at all.

Leading this research is Dr. Ajay Goel, the best person in the world to write a book on curcumin and cancer. This book can save your life!

Welcome to the 21st century of the healing arts, as healthcare grows to the next exciting level!

—Jacob Teitelbaum, M.D.
Author of *The Fatigue and Fibromyalgia Solution, From Fatigued to Fantastic, Beating Sugar Addiction, Real Cause, Real Cure,* and *Pain Free 1-2-3*

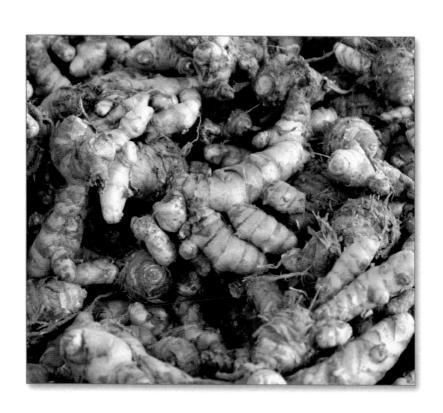

PART 1

Curcumin and Cancer

CHAPTER 1

Why We're Losing the War on Cancer

The U.S. declared war on cancer more than 50 years ago. We're losing that war.

More than $100 billion has been spent on cancer research in the U.S. alone, resulting in a host of outrageously expensive and largely ineffective new drugs and implementing cutting edge diagnostic techniques. Despite this enormous expenditure, the cancer death rate, adjusted for the size and age of the population, has only decreased by 5% since 1950, according to a 2009 *New York Times* article.

If you have cancer, if you know anyone with cancer or if anyone you love has died of cancer, you might be feeling angry right now. Your anger would be well justified.

Why are we losing the war on cancer?

I'll give you a simple answer: We're losing the war on cancer because we did not recognize that each person's cancer is a unique and individual disease. There is no one-size-fits-all solution. Cancer is a terribly complex disease.

What's more, laser-targeted approaches to cancer treatment will inevitably fail because cancer cells are smart. They're so smart that they almost seem to have a brain. As soon as we target cancer cells from one direction, they change direction and become resistant to whatever therapy worked last week or last month.

To successfully treat cancer, we must first understand the individual nature of each person's cancer. Then we must approach that cancer from a wide variety of ways. We need to *see* what will work this week and *anticipate* what will work next week, because what will work in the future course of an individual's disease will assuredly be different than what has worked in the past.

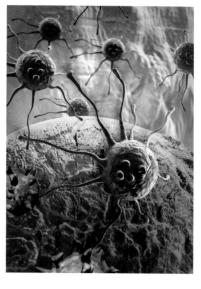

You already know this is a book on curcumin. There will be a lot more detail on curcumin and how it works, but ponder this as we proceed:

> **Curcumin is one of the only naturally occurring medicines known to science that targets cancer from so many directions at once.**

I say this without qualification. Curcumin is a natural substance and it is one of the only substances, natural or synthetic, that science has proven addresses and combats cancer in so many different ways.

Failure of the War on Cancer

Let's take a moment to go back and look at the War on Cancer. I said at the beginning of this chapter that our net gain against cancer in the last 65 years is a paltry 5%.

We've made great strides against many other diseases.

Since 1950, we've cut heart disease deaths by more than

60%. We've slashed the number of deaths from strokes by two-thirds and deaths from pneumonia and influenza are less than half what they were at mid-century. Yet our progress against cancer has been minimal.

The cancer death rate has remained virtually unchanged since 1950. In fact, cancer deaths are projected to increase by 30% from 7 million a year in 2002 to 10 million in 2020. Those figures, also adjusted for age and population, rise to a truly frightening 14 million a year by 2030—doubling the 2002 death rate.

Extrapolate the millions upon millions of cancer deaths since 1950, and it's easy to understand why every doctor, medical researcher, cancer patient, and cancer patient's family has every right to feel angry and frustrated.

President Richard Nixon declared war on cancer in his 1971 State of the Union address, vowing to "conquer this dread disease (and make the United States) . . . become the healthiest nation in the world."

Between 1997 and 2008, several targeted anticancer drugs

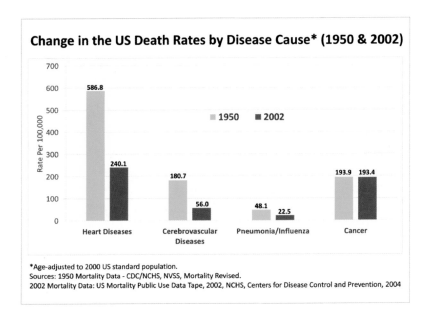

Change in the US Death Rates by Disease Cause* (1950 & 2002)

*Age-adjusted to 2000 US standard population.
Sources: 1950 Mortality Data - CDC/NCHS, NVSS, Mortality Revised.
2002 Mortality Data: US Mortality Public Use Data Tape, 2002, NCHS, Centers for Disease Control and Prevention, 2004

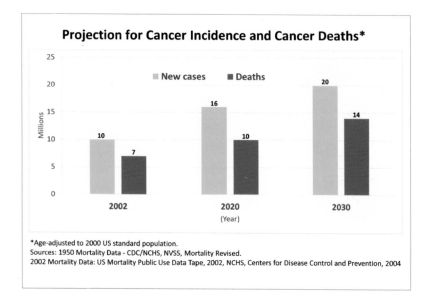

Projection for Cancer Incidence and Cancer Deaths*

*Age-adjusted to 2000 US standard population.
Sources: 1950 Mortality Data - CDC/NCHS, NVSS, Mortality Revised.
2002 Mortality Data: US Mortality Public Use Data Tape, 2002, NCHS, Centers for Disease Control and Prevention, 2004

have been approved by the FDA, broadening the arsenal against a wide range of cancers, including breast, colorectal, multiple myeloma and prostate, some costing as much as $300,000 for one year's treatment, not to speak of surgeries, transplants and associated expenses that can bankrupt a family.

All for nothing.

Yes, there are indeed cases where lives are saved or prolonged with treatment, but at the same time, when you consider the numbers as a whole, we are making very little progress.

The best cancer patients and their families can hope for with some of these "exciting" new drugs is at best a handful of months or weeks of life made miserable by the terrible side effects. In fact, one drug that costs $144,000 a year can be expected to add only six weeks to a colorectal cancer patient's life.

Every single one of these expensive drugs has a single target or addresses a single cancer pathway.

I have been researching cancer for more than 20 years. I can say unequivocally that cancer is a different disease in every single case.

Yes, there are commonalities that I will address, but cancer involves a complex roadmap of genes and pathways that can take on exponential numbers of possibilities. Therefore, we need to approach it knowing that those smart cancer cells can adapt to the ever-evolving disease in each cancer patient with impressive speed.

Cancer commonalities

Many people think that cancer is hereditary. Everyone can tell you the story of colon cancer or breast cancer that "runs in families."

Yes, the Genome Project has opened many doors, including helping us define the exact genomes that can cause cancer.

That has led to the discovery that heredity alone causes cancer in less than 5% of all cases.

If cancer or heart disease or Alzheimer's or any of these terrible diseases "run in" your family, the underlying cause is seldom what most of us would think.

These are diseases of Western civilization that are rarely the result of a hand of fate dealt by some nebulous "bad genes."

Most cancers have their origins in lifestyle choices and the environment. These are the choices that "run in families," ranging from diet or alcohol and tobacco consumption, exercise habits, stress management and where we live, play and work every day of our lives.

We have also inherited the dietary and lifestyle choices made by our parents and grandparents, not an inherited propensity for cancer or any other disease.

Cancer and the other dread diseases are almost entirely caused by eating too much, eating the wrong foods and living in an industrialized society that is poisoning our earth, air, water and food.

We have control over some of these choices and for some, such as the polluted air we breathe or the tainted water from municipal systems, we do not.

And yes, genes do play a role here. Our lifestyle choices can turn off cancer-preventing genes and turn on cancer-promoting genes in the blink of an eye. Self-destructive lifestyle choices not only affect us as individuals, they directly affect the gene structures of our children and their children and their children . . .

Generational choices

Have you ever considered that what you put in your mouth, whether you are a man or a woman, directly affects the life of your unborn child and creates a risk for a lifetime of pain, disease and early death?

I know it sounds grim, but stay with me here.

A comprehensive study of food availability of Swedish families as far back as the 1890s showed that fathers who were somewhat food deprived around puberty passed on a resistance to cardiovascular disease in their children. Conversely, children and grandchildren of those who had abundant food during the same period in their lives had an increased risk of death from diabetes.

"These findings suggest that diet can cause changes to genes that are passed down through generations by the males in a family, and that these alterations can affect susceptibility to certain diseases," wrote lead researcher Daniel Simmons, Ph.D., director of cancer research at Brigham Young University.

It's a sobering train of thought and one that should give all of us more reason to reconsider our lifestyle decisions.

An ounce of prevention

Without a doubt, it's better to prevent cancer or any disease than to treat it.

Of course, you might ask, "How do you know when you didn't get cancer (or heart disease or diabetes or Alzheimer's)?"

You don't. You can never know the cancer you didn't get or the heart attack you didn't have. But we do know that people who engage in healthy lifestyles have much lower rates of cancer, heart disease and more.

This book is primarily based on my own research on curcumin and cancer, but it is impossible to separate the underlying causes of cancer from the causes of other diseases, especially inflammation and epigenetics. We'll go into those in great detail in the coming chapters.

Most of my research has focused on colorectal cancer, one of the most common cancers in the U.S. and in many Western countries.

Here's what we've learned about colorectal cancer that has far-reaching implications for the prevention and treatment of other diseases:

Today we can assure a 90% cure rate for colorectal cancers detected early. Yes, that means we need colonoscopies until something better comes along. I know you all hate them, but they're worth it! For those whose cancers are diagnosed in the later stages, 3 and 4, fewer than 5% of those with colon cancer will survive for five years.

And here's the key: Colorectal cancer is almost exclusively a lifestyle disease. It is the only cancer that is truly preventable with proper diet.

And another important point: Colorectal cancer is 10 to 15 times more common in the "developed" world, but when people from Second and Third World countries migrate to the Western world, their ethnic protection against colorectal cancer disappears in as little as one generation—all because of the Western processed meat and potatoes diet.

What can you do about it?

These dire statistics are daunting to all of us.

Let me begin by assuring you that there is a great deal you can do to prevent cancer, heart disease, diabetes and many other dread diseases. There is much you can do even if you've already been diagnosed with one or more of these diseases.

Please understand that you and your family are not to blame for your health challenges. There is no point in pointing fingers.

What's more, I'm not urging you to become an anti-Monsanto activist or even a vegetarian or vegan, although there is a lot to be said for all three.

Instead, I'm asking you to become aware of your lifestyle and the choices you make that vastly increase your risk of cancer and several other chronic diseases that we'll address in the coming chapters.

Here are some of the biggest choices we all have to make, the ones that can have the greatest effect on our health and the health of our offspring.

1. **Eat meat? Be a vegetarian or vegan?** This is a very personal decision. Personally, I don't think it is really a problem if you consume small amounts of organic meat or dairy products. The problem is really in the hormones and antibiotics and GMO-modified feed that pollute most non-organic meat and milk. In my native India, many people consume several glasses of milk a day with no apparent harmful effects, largely because growth hormones and antibiotics are not given to the cows to increase milk production in India and cattle are not raised on GMO-tainted feed. It's important to make the choice to eat organic as much as possible and to

avoid processed foods and GMO (genetically modified organism) foods, including almost all soy and corn products.

2. **Overeating.** Dozens of studies show that caloric restriction results in longer life and less chronic disease. In the U.S., people are large and, let me be honest, sometimes obese. Food is abundant and cheap and frequently of low nutritional quality. We eat far more than we need or than we should. I think this nation of obese people is actually starving for the nutrients we so desperately need that are not available in our food. We think we need more protein than we do and we get too much from hormone-laced animal sources, which increases the risk of cancer. Research shows organic meats and dairy products are less risky, but protein from vegetable sources is totally safe and does not promote cancer growth. Dried beans are an excellent low-fat source of protein, fiber, B vitamins, iron, magnesium and other minerals. Just cutting 500–700 calories from your calorie intake can have profound effects on your longevity and your risk of cancer.

There are many factors that influence overweight and obesity, including food additives. Even though it may be difficult to lose all the weight you wish, it is never too late to start eating healthier, with more fresh, unprocessed foods. This in turn may help you start to lose weight naturally.

3. **Reducing toxic load.** We live in a toxic world. The degree to which we are exposed to poisons is truly horrifying. We are barraged with toxins every day of our lives. Every morning, we shampoo with carcinogenic products, slather on moisturizer laced with cancer-causing chemicals, put on deodorant and brush our teeth with products known to cause breast cancer and then put on our petrochemical-based clothing to face the toxic work world where we breathe in off-gassing synthetic carpets, fumes from fiber board furniture saturated in formaldehyde, and recycled air.

While some toxic exposure is out of your control, there are a few important choices you can make to minimize this exposure that can reap major benefits, including using organic personal care products, installing a whole house water filter and controlling the use of pesticides and herbicides on your own property. Simply removing your shoes at the door is a huge step in minimizing toxic chemicals you might track in from the outside world into your home.

Other diseases

The numbers aren't much more encouraging for other deadly diseases. The World Health Organization projects that 23.3 million people worldwide will die of heart disease each year by 2030, compared to 17.3 million in 2008. In the U.S., about 600,000 people die of heart disease each year and 42 million of us are living with some form of heart disease. Then there's diabetes. More than 19.7 million Americans have been diagnosed with diabetes and another 8.2 million have the disease but don't know it. Add on an astronomical 50.7 million more who have pre-diabetes and you begin to get a picture of the seriousness of the diabetes problem alone.

I'm throwing this endless array of numbers at you for a reason.

Folks, these are *all* lifestyle diseases.

Yes, your grandfather may have died of a heart attack at age 50 and your mother and grandmother and you may have diabetes, but the genetic component of those diseases is miniscule. This is all about choices you can make right now to minimize your risk of cancer, heart disease, diabetes and other diseases, awaken those disease-fighting genes that have gone to sleep and restore your body to the healthy balance that is your birthright.

The good news

With all of these dire statistics, it might seem easy to sink down on the couch with a quart of ice cream and give up trying.

Nothing could be farther from the right path.

Many of the factors, genetic, epigenetic and environmental, are reversible. Let me repeat that to be sure you get the message very clearly:

Most of these changes are reversible.

You have the power to choose the right diet, right exercise, right lifestyle and, most importantly, right supplementation to protect yourself from these dread diseases and more.

Not only are these effects reversible, it is never too late to change. Even if you've degenerated into a couch potato, poor eating habit kind of lifestyle, you can start reaping the benefits of genes that are awake, alive and alert at any time in your life. You can take steps to stop the destructive force of inflammation.

Of course, change doesn't happen overnight, so don't wait until you have a problem. Prevention is always the best course.

How does curcumin fit into this picture?

If you love curry, you'll be familiar with turmeric, a popular, vividly colored golden spice.

Turmeric in itself has a plethora of health benefits, if you're willing to eat it in huge quantities from childhood on. Botanically known as *Curcuma longa,* the turmeric rhizome is a member of the antioxidant-rich ginger family.

You might be understandably skeptical when you hear that this humble Indian spice can prevent, treat and sometimes even cure a wide variety of serious diseases. These include everything from cancer, heart disease, the pain of all types of arthritis and even "incurable" diseases like diabetes and

Alzheimer's. Curcumin has shown positive effects in treating every single disease for which it has been studied.

For centuries, this super plant has given the gift of long life and robust health to my ancestors in India, for whom various types of curries—always made with turmeric—are a dietary staple eaten several times a day.

It is also an integral part of religious traditions in the Indian Hindu culture. Its golden paste applied to the forehead is used in devotional ceremonies and weddings.

For more than 6,000 years, turmeric has been used as a medicine in one of the oldest systems of traditional medicine, Ayurveda, which seeks to bring balance to the body's elemental substances and energy centers. Recent research shows that most of the benefits attributed to turmeric in the Ayurvedic tradition actually come from curcumin. It is sometimes called "the Golden Goddess" because of its vast healing powers.

Now we get down to the 21st century practical application:

Inside turmeric is a compound called curcumin, which is

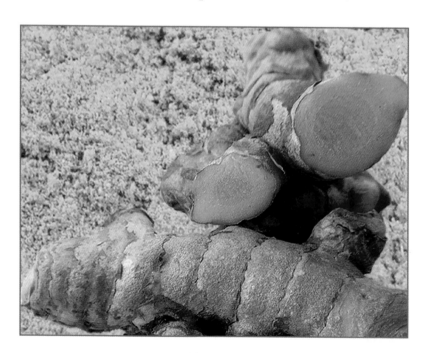

found in its rhizome (the stem of the plant found underground). Curcumin is responsible for the golden orange color of turmeric, and is perhaps the most powerful naturally occurring medicine known to humankind today. In simple terms, turmeric is the spice and curcumin is the medicine.

Curcumin has shown positive effects in treating every single disease for which it has been studied.

However, there is very little curcumin in the spice turmeric. If you've seen cheap turmeric supplements on the market, understand that they only contain 2 to 5% curcumin, which may or may not be usable by your body. They're not likely to have much effectiveness in terms of prevention or treatment for the diseases we're talking about. Curcumin is *many times* more powerful than turmeric.

In the 21st century, curcumin's medicinal value is backed by voluminous research that credits its healing powers to its exceptional antioxidant and anti-inflammatory properties.

Curcumin is by far one of the most powerful antioxidants known to science, hundreds of times more powerful than blueberries, which have substantial antioxidant capabilities themselves.

Curcumin literally scrubs the oxidative "rust" from your cells, preventing serious disease and reversing diseases you may already have. It helps stop cell deterioration and restores cellular genetic codes to youthful levels, ensuring those cells will reproduce more like they did when you were young.

On the ORAC (Oxygen Radical Absorbance Capacity) scale that rates the antioxidant power of foods, the antioxidant power of the more bioavailable preparations of curcumin rate over 15,000 per 1 *single* gram, while antioxidant-rich blueberries have only a 600 ORAC rating per single gram! This means that just one high-quality curcumin capsule delivers more than 25 times the antioxidants as the same amount of blueberries.

We'll learn more about the connection between inflammation and cancer in the next chapter, but let it suffice to say here that curcumin's antioxidant superpowers result in lower levels of inflammation and lower risk of cancer and a host of other chronic diseases.

More important, from the viewpoint of damaged cell division found in cancer, curcumin also tells these cells to die when their time comes, as ordained by nature, which stops tumor growth. It also helps kill cancerous tumors by cutting off their blood supply, stops the spread of cancer and kills cancer stem cells that stay alive in your bloodstream for years, preventing recurrences of old cancers. It even enhances the effectiveness of chemotherapy drugs and radiation therapy commonly used in conventional cancer treatment.

WHAT YOU NEED TO KNOW

* Cancer diagnosis and death rates have not changed significantly in the past 40 years, despite earlier detection techniques. This means that more cancers are occurring, probably because of our lifestyle and environment.

* Your lifestyle, particularly your eating choices, are the most powerful predictors of your lifelong health, your risk of cancer, heart disease, and the other commonly recognized "diseases of aging."

* Overeating is probably our greatest controllable health risk.

* We can change our risk of cancer by controlling environmental factors and lifestyle choices.

* Curcumin fights cancer in a variety of powerful ways, making it our most potent weapon against this disease.

CHAPTER 2

Cancer Is an Inflammatory Disease

Cancer is almost exclusively a lifestyle disease. By that, I'm not vesting blame on anyone, but I am reminding you that we all make choices about our lifestyles and that each of us can step up and make positive choices whenever possible.

You may not be able to control the off-gassing carpets and formaldehyde-laden fiberboard furniture in your office or in a public building, but you *can* choose what you put in your own home.

You may not be able to control whether your neighbor sprays RoundUp™ in his yard, but you can choose the types of weed control you use on your own property.

You may not be able to control the food you are served when you're eating in restaurants, while you're on vacation or on a business trip, but you choose what you serve in your own home.

It's interesting that the Western world has by far the highest cancer rates. It's also fascinating that cancer rates have skyrocketed in Japan since the 1950s, when the traditional cancer preventive diet was abandoned for the modern, Western diet with an accompanying cancer rate comparable to that in the Western world.

Common underlying cause

Cancer can be caused by any (or several) of a wide variety of things, but inflammation is definitely one of the major culprits in almost all chronic illnesses, including cancer. Inflammation triggers a cascade of events that lead to virtually every type of cancer.

Let's be sure we're on the same page here:

If you've ever whacked your thumb with a hammer or sprained your ankle, you have experienced acute inflammation—often characterized by redness, swelling, bruising and pain. The immune system sends out its warriors—white blood cells—to neutralize such inflammatory stress. It hurts for a while, maybe requiring a little pain medicine or ice, and then

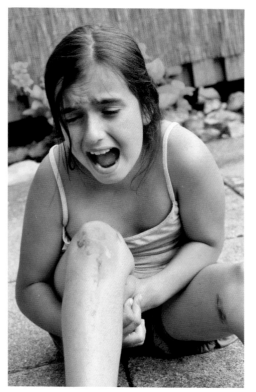

it's gone. The body heals itself and there is no lasting damage. Controlled inflammation is your body's natural response to an injury.

In contrast however, chronic inflammation is another thing altogether. Low-level chronic inflammation is an excessive and inappropriate inflammatory response. It is a silent killer that may have no symptoms at all. It often goes completely unnoticed.

Acute inflammation has visible symptoms and can usually be controlled by pain relievers and anti-inflammatory drugs. Chronic inflammation has no symptoms and must be managed by safe, non-toxic medicines, like curcumin.

Let's go back to some biology basics here. I promise they won't be painful.

The human immune system helps defend cells and tissues from outside attacks. It fights infection and handles attacks from anything it perceives as a foreign invader. Those foreign invaders can take a wide variety of forms, including bacterial, viral or fungal infections. In general, these invaders are environmental: they are the things you put in and on your body, the air you breathe, and the water you drink.

These "invaders" (think of them as unwelcome visitors) can trigger a low level of inflammation, that can last for a long time, even decades. If it continues unchecked, it disrupts several biological functions, including the all-important immune system.

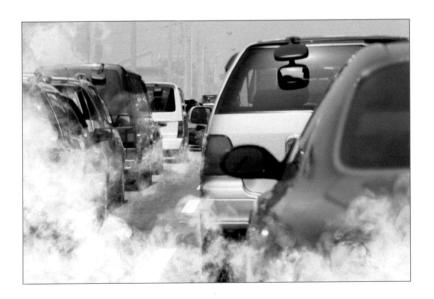

Chronic inflammation is caused by the same lifestyle choices we talked about in Chapter 1:

- eating processed and adulterated foods

- overeating

- smoking

- breathing polluted air

- drinking municipal water

- using toxic personal care products (shampoo, soap, toothpaste, makeup, deodorant and more)

- toxic cleaning products

- petrochemicals and gas fumes

- pesticides and herbicides

- living and working in toxic environments (off-gassing carpets, furniture and bedding)

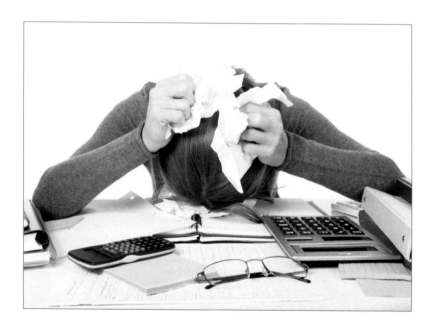

If you are obese, or have diabetes, heart disease, Alzheimer's, osteoporosis, depression or cancer, you have a disease triggered by chronic inflammation. If you don't have any of these diseases yet, count yourself lucky, be proactive about it, and do what you can to prevent or minimize things that lead to low-level inflammation.

Chronic inflammation puts you at high risk for an array of diseases. All of us need to be worried about it.

The role of chronic stress in inflammation

Long-term unrelieved stress is another important cause of chronic inflammation. Who doesn't experience stress on a daily, perhaps even hourly basis these days? Sometimes we don't even recognize it, but we are actually stressed about the small day-to-day, stuff, like getting kids to school, meeting a work deadline or getting stuck in traffic. Each of these stressors can trigger chronic inflammation.

The human body is designed to respond to threats with a cascade of biological events that give us superhuman strength.

Imagine this: Your child has wandered into the street. You feel that surge of adrenaline. You run faster than you ever imagined possible. You dart between cars, heart pounding, your brain laser focused and hyper alert. When you finally grab onto the precious little one, you exhale a huge sigh of relief, unaware that you had been holding your breath. When you finally bring her to safety, you sink to the ground, relieved and exhausted.

Without being aware of it, you've just demonstrated the instinctive stress and release response ingrained in the human race since the beginning of our species.

Biologically, when there is an acute stress situation, your adrenal glands release a flood of adrenaline, cortisol and other chemicals that shut down every bodily system that is not needed for survival in the next few minutes. Digestion has slowed. Wound healing is put on hold. Your liver has released stored glucose for energy.

So just like acute inflammation that we discussed a few pages back, saving your child from traffic is a threat that has a beginning, middle and an end. It takes place in a few seconds, a minute at most.

Our ancestors dealt with frequent life-threatening situations. Most of these crises ended with a time of relaxation and relief.

Now let's switch gears to today's world. We rarely experience life-threatening events, yet stress just keeps piling on us, unrelieved, hour after hour, day after day. While you might not often feel the heart-pounding superhuman powers of the threat of your child wandering in traffic, your body is responding in exactly the same way, even if the threat is only your child's poor grade on a test, a looming deadline at work, or an argument with your spouse.

And—here's the important part—we don't take the recovery time our bodies and minds desperately need. Voila! Chronic stress. And chronic stress is the mother of chronic inflammation.

What happens when you have chronic inflammation?

I've already mentioned that chronic inflammation compromises the healthy immune system, among the many destructive effects it has on the human body.

It also causes the production of free radical oxygen molecules, which damage the DNA of cells. The DNA is a blueprint on how to make a new cell. If the blueprint is damaged, the new cell is defective. It may even be mutated into a cancer cell.

These inflammatory triggers—perceived as foreign invaders by your immune system—start a slow cascade that opens you up to a variety of diseases.

A strong, healthy immune system can easily handle an invader, whether it's the flu virus or even the occasional fast food attack. But over a lifetime, the foreign invaders begin to pile on and your immune system weakens.

Then these invaders begin to search for weak points, and gradually they find a way to cause mutations in critical genes. Your weakened immune system is a defense mechanism with no way to repair the damage to one or two or several thousand genes, or even to millions of cells, so they continue to multiply. The seed is sown.

Many things begin to go awry.

Every cell has a definite lifespan, and this process is very efficiently regulated by *apoptosis* or programmed cell death. A compromised immune system can affect the genes that control such death signals. Cells that don't get those death signals live on and on, far beyond their normal lifespan. New cells continue to be born, while the old cells don't die, so the cells continue to pile up in large masses. This old-cell logjam essentially leads to the formation of tumors and cancers. In other words, cancers can simply be viewed as abnormal growth of otherwise normal cells.

> Cancer is an abnormal growth of otherwise normal cells
> that fail to die, become immortal and continue
> to pile up, creating tumors.

The old-cell logjam doesn't necessarily always lead to formation of cancer, but it can have other effects in other parts of the body as well. For example, if old cells become rooted in the pancreas, they can interrupt the natural renewal of islet cells, eventually damaging the body's ability to produce insulin and causing diabetes. In the brain, the inflammation can impair the function of neurons and result in Alzheimer's disease.

Cancer cells are incredibly smart. I am well aware that it is not scientifically sound, but it's almost like these evil little creatures have brains. They thwart virtually every type of treatment we try. They shuffle nutrients away from other parts of the body and divert blood supplies for their own growth. They even grow new blood vessels to feed themselves and ensure their survival, a process called *angiogenesis.*

NF-Kappa B is one of the most important cellular factors that controls inflammation inside cells. It is the hub of inflammation. Without going into deep scientific explanation, it's important to know that NF-Kappa B is an inflammation-causing protein that is intimately linked to the way hundreds of other genes eventually behave. In most healthy cells, NF-Kappa-B levels are very tightly controlled. But sometimes, it becomes overactive and upsets the inflammatory balance, almost like an allergic reaction. Eventually, the long-term inflammation triggered by NF-Kappa B hyperactivity can cause and promote cancer.

Deadly drugs to combat chronic inflammation

Can't we just take some sort of drug to combat chronic inflammation?

I wish the answer was that easy, but sadly, it's not.

You've no doubt heard of NSAIDs—non-steroidal anti-inflammatory drugs. That's just scientific jargon for drugs used to treat inflammation, fever, and pain. This includes over-the-counter medicines like aspirin, ibuprofen and naproxen (Aleve) as well as prescription medicines like celecoxib (Celebrex), piroxicam (Feldene), diclofenac (Cambia, Cataflam, Voltaren and more), oxaprozin (Daypro) and several others.

These drugs, prescription or not, belong to a class called cyclooxygenase or COX 1 and 2-enzyme pathway inhibitors, which are intended to block inflammation. I won't drag you through a complicated scientific explanation for all of that except to say that these are systems that should not be disrupted or blocked.

There are several serious health consequences for people taking these drugs, some of them even caused by short-term use:

- Doubled risk of heart attack and stroke

- Doubled risk of death from heart attack or stroke

- Gastrointestinal bleeding, sometimes fatal

- Gastric ulcers

- Kidney failure

- Liver failure

- Blood thinning leading to prolonged bleeding after surgery or injury

In fact, as many as 16,500 deaths each year are attributed to the gastrointestinal complications of long-term use of the NSAID ibuprofen in the U.S. alone. That number climbs to 30,000 when you combine all the NSAIDs.

It is simply not safe to take these drugs every day to relieve chronic inflammation, even though doctors commonly prescribe these drugs and you can find them on any drug store shelf.

Please avoid them and talk to your doctor about your desire to avoid their use whenever possible.

WHAT YOU NEED TO KNOW

◆ Chronic inflammation is a silent killer with no symptoms.

◆ Lifestyle choices, especially dietary choices, obesity and unmanaged stress, cause chronic inflammation.

◆ Stress is a major factor in creating chronic inflammation.

◆ This type of inflammation is a trigger for cancer, diabetes, Alzheimer's disease and many of the common diseases of aging.

◆ Chronic inflammation disrupts the immune system, leading to cell damage that allows uncontrolled cell reproduction and cancer.

◆ Anti-inflammatory drugs may actually worsen the problem.

◆ Long-term use of NSAIDs should be avoided, as these are not an answer to reduce chronic inflammation.

CHAPTER 3

Curcumin–Getting Back to Our Roots

Curcumin has shown positive effects for every single disease for which it has been studied.

Its anti-inflammatory, antioxidant, antimicrobial and anti-cancer properties are unique in the plant world. That's what makes curcumin the ideal botanical medicine to conquer virtually every type of cancer and many chronic diseases.

Clearly, nobody wants to have cancer. Without doubt, preventing cancer through a healthy diet and lifestyle is preferable, especially in view of the ineffectiveness and toxicity of the anticancer drugs currently on the market. Curcumin is an excellent preventive, as well as one of the most powerful tools we currently have to prevent and treat cancer. In fact, it is validated by more than 8,000 published, peer-reviewed, scientific articles.

So what is curcumin? If you love curry, you're no doubt familiar with turmeric, the vivid orange-colored spice that gives curry its distinctive flavor. Inside turmeric is a compound called curcumin, perhaps the most powerful botanical medicine known to mankind.

However, as healthy as turmeric is as a spice, it has a very low curcumin content. Unless you were born into a culture that consumes turmeric-laden meals three times a day as part of your daily diet for your entire life, you're unlikely to get any real health or medicinal benefit from consuming an occasional meal containing this tasty spice.

The curcumin content of turmeric is only 2 to 5%, depending upon the species of turmeric, and the climate and soil where it is grown in different parts of the world. Although turmeric may be the most natural way of achieving health benefits of curcumin, such an approach is not practical for those who can't consume enough turmeric on a daily basis for a lifetime. That's why turmeric is not likely to be anywhere close to as effective as curcumin for prevention or treatment for cancer or the other diseases we're talking about. Curcumin is *many times* more powerful than turmeric.

Turmeric is the spice and curcumin is the medicine.

Turmeric is the healthy spice.
Curcumin is the natural medicine present in turmeric.

This humble herb, used in India for millennia, has no known serious side effects and no toxicity, even when taken in large amounts.

Turmeric has been an integral part of the religious traditions and customs of India's predominantly Hindu culture for more than 6,000 years. My compatriots in India eat large

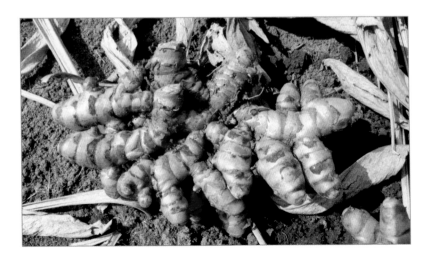

amounts of turmeric several times every day in their favorite curry dishes.

Cancer rates in India are very low, probably due to the universal consumption of turmeric and other medicinal herbs and spices people eat as part of their daily diet several times a day for a lifetime. Fewer than 1 million cases of cancer were reported in India in 2010 in a population of 1.2 billion. That means cancer is rare, striking only one in every 12,000 people in India. Compare that to the shockingly high U.S. cancer rate. The lifetime cancer risk for an American man is 50% and 33% for women. In simple terms, the cancer rate in the U.S. is 30 times higher than in India.

They're certainly doing something right in India, although it's interesting to note that the cancer rate is projected to increase in the coming years, in part due to the increasing popularity of Westernized diets. I have no doubt that the traditional Indian diet has provided protection against cancer and other dread diseases. If my compatriots would continue to eat a traditional diet, I have no doubt their cancer protection would remain in place.

We've talked about the destructive effects of chronic inflammation. I'll add here that curcumin is one of the most potent anti-inflammatory botanical substances known to science.

Curcumin: the anti-inflammatory powerhouse

Curcumin works as an anti-inflammatory to prevent the growth of cancerous cells in a variety of ways.

1. It inhibits the COX-2 and NF-Kappa B inflammatory pathways, preventing chronic inflammation.

2. It scrubs away the free radical oxygen molecules that promote the growth of arachidonic acid, a hormone that has been called "the mother of inflammation."

3. It controls the body's production of cytokines, proteins that serve as molecular messengers between cells. When there are too many pro-inflammatory cytokines, chronic inflammation is the ultimate consequence.

4. It slows or stops the production of certain enzymes, such as protein kinases, that increase inflammation.

If all of this science is a bit confusing, not to worry. It's just important to know that curcumin works in these distinctly different, but powerful ways, to stop chronic inflammation that have been linked to cancer and other diseases commonly associated with the aging process. This means that cancer can't get a foothold. Without chronic inflammation, there is no distorted reproduction of damaged cells that can eventually turn into cancer cells.

Antioxidant punch

Curcumin is also by far one of the most powerful antioxidants known to science, hundreds of times more powerful than blueberries and dark chocolate, which have substantial antioxidant capabilities themselves.

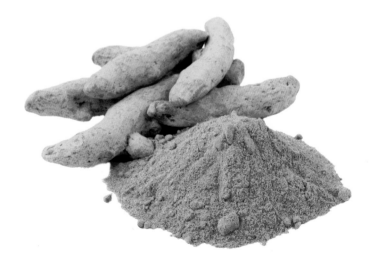

Curcumin literally scrubs the oxidative "rust" from your cells, preventing serious disease and reversing diseases you may already have. It helps stop cell deterioration and restores cellular genetic codes to more youthful levels, ensuring those cells will reproduce more like they did when you were young, which helps to prevent cancer and many other diseases associated with aging.

On the ORAC (Oxygen Radical Absorbance Capacity) scale that rates the antioxidant power of foods, the higher absorption preparation of curcumin, BCM-95™, has been shown to possess over 15,000 in one single gram, while antioxidant-rich blueberries have only a 600 ORAC rating per gram. The BCM-95™ form of curcumin is one of the most clinically studied high absorption types of curcumin in the world.

Of course, this doesn't mean you shouldn't eat blueberries; they contain a vast variety of healthy nutrients. What this means is that just one high-quality curcumin capsule delivers more than 25 times the antioxidants as the same amount of blueberries.

Curcumin's broad-based attack against cancer

In the coming chapters, we'll examine the multitude of ways that cancer cells are created, survive and thrive. We'll talk about:

Epigenetics: A process that controls the behavior of our genes, our genetics. Dietary and lifestyle choices and exposure to toxins can alter the way our genes work. For example, they can cause some protective genes to go to sleep and may cause destructive genes to wake up. When this happens, diseases can take hold.

Apoptosis: The programmed life cycle of cells. This natural cycle can be interrupted by a variety of causes. When cells don't die as nature intends, old and genetically flawed cells form tumors.

Angiogenesis: Cancer cells need nutrients and oxygen to survive, so they are able to create their own network of blood vessels, ensuring their survival.

Cancer stem cells: Super cells that govern other cancer cells and can remain dormant, sometimes for years, eventually causing cancer to recur.

Chemo-resistance: Cancer cells have the ability to evolve quickly and become resistant to chemotherapy treatments.

Chemo enhancement and radio enhancement: The ability of certain substances to sensitize and enhance the effectiveness of conventional chemotherapy and radiation therapies for cancer.

This is just the barest thumbnail explanation of the wide variety of ways that cancer takes hold in the human body.

As you can see, cancer is a tremendously complex disease. The present generation of anticancer drugs is designed to target a single gene or pathway within cancer cells, meaning each one approaches cancer in just one way. These mono-targeted drugs are the most commonly used conventional cancer treatments. They are largely ineffective precisely because they address only one small facet of cancer. They target one very small part of the complex network of hundreds of genes and pathways that cancer cells use for their survival, allowing those smart cancer cells to outsmart the drugs.

It is unlikely that we can successfully treat most cancers with drugs. Furthermore, virtually all conventional cancer drugs are outrageously expensive and only minimally effective. Increasingly, scientists have begun to realize that cancer can only be conquered if it is addressed from many directions.

That is why scientists have gone to great lengths to isolate active molecules (or medicines) from natural plant-based compounds. Nearly 75% of all approved anticancer drugs are derived from natural plant-based compounds or mimic certain aspects of the plant one way or another. As an aside, approximately 25% of all prescription drugs used in the U.S. are derived from plants.

However, these drugs, even the ones based on plants, are developed to address single-target pathways. Natural plant-based compounds, like curcumin, have the ability to target not just one gene or pathway, but to simultaneously control many different pathways. Such multi-targeted therapies attack cancer cells from many directions all at once and reduce their ability to survive and thrive.

Curcumin is one such compound that has been validated in thousands of scientific studies. Though other botanical medicines have been tested and a few have some multi-targeting properties, none compare to the strength of curcumin and its ability to address so many cancer genetic pathways at one time. This wide-ranging approach is far more effective in combatting this complex disease than the mono-targeted, modern, designer, chemotherapeutic drugs conventional medicine has unsuccessfully used for the past several decades.

In any case, if you have cancer, you should be working very closely with a trusted oncologist to determine all treatment approaches that are best for you. This includes the use of both modern and traditional options that are scientifically proven to help patients. If your physician is not familiar with the health benefits of curcumin and other complementary and alternative treatment medicines, educate your doctor about it. (See Chapter 13 for a synopsis of this book that I welcome you to print and give to your doctor.)

Have a meaningful and open discussion about the wealth of scientific evidence that has been published on the anticancer benefits of curcumin individually, and its use in conjunction with conventional cancer treatments.

I think this is the most natural route for conventional doctors to recognize curcumin as a bona fide treatment option for various diseases, including cancer.

WHAT YOU NEED TO KNOW

◆ Curcumin has shown positive effects for virtually every disease for which it has been studied.

◆ Curcumin is the most potent anti-inflammatory botanical known to science. It also has one of the highest antioxidant ratings of any food.

◆ Its anticancer properties are unique in the plant world and make it the ideal plant compound to conquer virtually every type of cancer and many chronic diseases.

◆ Curcumin attacks cancer from several directions ("multi-targeting"), making it potentially even more effective than drugs currently in use in conventional cancer treatment.

◆ Prevention is always preferable to treatment. A healthy diet and lifestyle are scientifically proven to prevent cancer. Curcumin can and should be part of a preventive lifestyle.

◆ Curcumin, by itself, or in conjunction with conventional treatment may be a powerful option for patients with various diseases, including cancer.

CHAPTER 4

Epigenetics: Awakening Sleeping Genes

Does cancer run in your family? Alzheimer's? Diabetes? Diseases that run in families are common, but you might be surprised to learn that these diseases are rarely hereditary.

Hereditary means a trait or feature has been passed from parent to child. Your blue eyes or curly hair or even your musical talent are all due to the genes you inherited from both of your parents. Heredity explains why cats always give birth to kittens and not puppies.

Less than 5% of all cases of cancer are hereditary, meaning just a few cancers are the result of damaged cells passed on from one generation to the next. This is good news because it means you have much more control over your cancer risk than perhaps you ever thought possible.

More than 95% of cancers are non-hereditary, or sporadic in nature. They occur as part of the aging process.

We are now recognizing that the majority of cancers are in fact largely influenced by the dietary and lifestyle choices we all make every single day and throughout our lifetimes. These factors have a profound impact on the 20,000-plus genes in our cells and determine the behavior of genes that control various behaviors, including cancer growth. In other words, as benign as it may seem, diet has a huge bearing on our risk of cancer and other dread diseases. Our eating habits also have a major influence over the genes that protect us from cancer.

For example, do you live in a culture that drinks green tea at every meal? That is cancer protective. Do you live in a culture where everyone smokes cigarettes? That increases cancer risk.

Epigenetics and your choices

Enter a relatively new field of science called epigenetics. This complex science can be explained relatively easily: Simply put, your diet and lifestyle influences how your genes work and dictates whether they are behaving well or poorly. Epigenetics explains the continuously changing behavior of our genes in response to various environments.

Everything your mother did before and during her pregnancy, everything you do from the day you are born, everything you eat, drink and are exposed to in your environment has an effect on your genes.

As you age and grow, it is natural that some of the genes may get turned off—or go to sleep—as a consequence of eating habits, exercise regimens and toxic environmental stresses. Other genes that encourage uncontrolled cell growth may get turned on, thus promoting cancer growth.

When you don't eat correctly or exercise regularly and you're exposed to toxins that are everywhere, including in the air we must all breathe and the water we must all drink, cancer-preventing genes can go to sleep on the job and allow diseases to get a foothold.

Unlike the small risk for hereditary cancers, cancer-related genes that are epigenetically controlled and are directly related to lifestyle choices are responsible for more than 95% of all cancers.

But here's the good news, in fact, the great news: Epigenetic changes are reversible. Unlike hereditary cancers where you have inherited a permanently defective gene, epigenetically affected genes can be easily corrected. Those changes can begin the moment you start making wiser lifestyle choices.

This is wonderful news. It highlights the promise that cancer is not our destiny. We actually have significant control of how our genes behave, as long as we are willing to make positive dietary and lifestyle choices.

> Epigenetic changes are reversible.
> The moment you start making wiser lifestyle choices,
> you can get back on track to a healthier life.

Damage to the genetic material in our cells is the root cause of many diseases, including cancer. It is certainly in everyone's best interest and within everyone's reach to keep our genomes healthy.

Making the right lifestyle choices has a profound effect on your genes' activity and your risk of cancer. Eating right and regularly consuming natural dietary botanicals and herbals, like curcumin, can be a very effective strategy for preventing cancer.

We inherit a set of genes from each of our parents, a combination of their genetic traits. Unless you are an identical twin, there will never be anyone else exactly like you. As you'll see in the coming pages, it's a giant lottery in which you have a great deal more control than just random luck.

Identical twins validate the science of epigenetics

I think the study of identical twins is the greatest argument for the validity of the newly emerging science of epigenetics. We can all agree that identical twins are genetically identical, right? Their DNA is identical.

Yet anyone who has known identical twins knows that as they grow and age, they begin to look different. Their body types may be different. In time, they begin to develop different lifestyles and different habits. And, over time, one may develop cancer or another of the chronic diseases we've been talking about while the other does not.

Why?

This is the simplest explanation of epigenetics: diet and lifestyle choices and exposure to toxins cause some protective genes to go to sleep and may cause destructive genes to wake up or go into overdrive. When this happens, diseases can take hold. This is why one identical twin might get cancer or diabetes while the other remains healthy.

In simple terms, the discovery of epigenetics helps us dispel the notion that, "Cancer is my destiny," or "Cancer cannot be prevented," simply because a family member may have had cancer. Epigenetics helps us understand that genetic or hereditary forms of most cancers are extremely rare and that most cancers can be realistically prevented or managed by making simple day-to-day changes in our diets.

> Cancer is not your destiny. Cancer can be prevented by making smart dietary and lifestyle choices.

Here's another way to look at it: Genetics and epigenetics can be compared to a computer system. Genetics is the hardware and epigenetics is the software. The computer hardware (your gene structure) doesn't change, but the software (the ability of genes to behave or misbehave) can be constantly improved to enhance the performance of the computer. You can even re-write that genetic software to correct broken genetic "codes," that may be giving wrong information to your cells, causing malfunctions.

My family history

My family history is an excellent example of epigenetics. I lost my father, grandfather, and grandmother to complications of diabetes. I can easily tell you that about 80% of the members of my extended family have Type 2 diabetes. Every time I return home for a visit, my relatives warn me to "be careful about diabetes" since it "runs in the family."

There is no question that my family is at particular risk for diabetes, not necessarily because of a genetic propensity, but because of our familial or maybe cultural eating patterns that cause those diabetes-repressing genes to malfunction.

I am proud of my Indian heritage, but our diet is extremely heavy in unhealthy white rice and fried foods. I rarely see Indian people who are extremely obese, but I see lots of lean people with big bellies. Our bone structure is meant to be lean like other Asians, but somehow some of us are able to stretch out our bellies by eating huge quantities of foods that make us vulnerable to Type 2 diabetes.

I'm very careful about what I eat and when I go back to India, I eat mostly vegetables and only a little bit of rice. Yes, I know I am at risk for diabetes and I am doing everything I can to keep my insulin-producing mechanisms functioning properly so my genes will not go to sleep. I do not intend to become a victim of the family diabetes problem. I am careful about my eating habits.

I know for sure that I have taken every possible step to prevent diabetes. I have taken control. I may die of a million other things, but most likely it won't be of diabetes or its complications because I have made the choices to keep my anti-diabetes genes awake.

Choosing a gene-friendly diet

It isn't just cultural heritage that causes genes to behave badly.

Dietary patterns all over the world are the underlying causes of cancer. The Standard American Diet (SAD) is probably the most insidious choice, considering the high rates of cancer and cancer deaths in the Western world. Heavy on processed foods, factory farm-raised meats and dairy products and light on fruits and vegetables, the SAD leaves hundreds of millions of people unnecessarily vulnerable to cancer and other chronic diseases. The SAD tells anticancer genes loud and clear that it is OK to go to sleep and wakes up the cancer-producing genes.

So how does epigenetics work in terms of other diseases, like diabetes, that is so prevalent in my family?

The pancreas contains insulin-producing cells. Insulin balances the glucose in our diets, hopefully from fruits and vegetables and grains. Probably in reality, more often the glucose in our diets comes from sugar, sweets, refined grains and processed foods.

If the genes that tell cells to produce insulin go to sleep, like in most people with diabetes, the pancreas doesn't produce enough insulin and sugars aren't neutralized, causing diabetes and wide-ranging health problems ranging from heart disease to kidney failure to amputations and blindness. By keeping those genes awake and telling pancreatic cells to produce insulin, we have the ability to prevent diabetes.

Once you make those diet and lifestyle changes, you have the ability to turn things around, to wake up these genes, and make them do what they are supposed to do. Even in those who have already been diagnosed with diabetes, such defective genes can be re-awakened and the degeneration caused by diabetes can be minimized. Whatever chronic disease we are considering, the right dietary choices can minimize the disease risk and, if you already have the disease, it may even be reversed. It's such an easy solution, and it's hard for me to see why more of us aren't running as fast as we can toward a healthier and leaner diet.

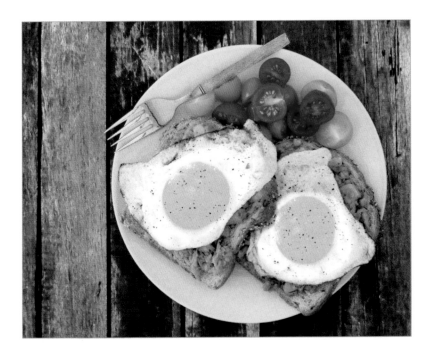

Epigenetics is a fundamentally fluid process. Everything about our health can change as soon as we make the right choices, allow our defective genes to reawaken and behave as they are supposed to when we were healthier.

To continue our computer analogy, we have tumor-suppressive genes whose job, like the anti-viral software on a computer, is to control the wild cell growth that results in cancer. We also have tumor-promoting genes that encourage out-of-control cell growth. Perfect health occurs when all these systems are perfectly balanced.

We already know that cells are programmed to be born, reproduce, and die on schedule. Anything that disrupts this life cycle can potentially cause wild cell growth and cancer.

Other factors

Diet isn't the only thing that may lull genes to sleep. For example, toxic exposures are definitely a serious problem.

In our increasingly toxic world, a wide variety of chemicals increase the risk of putting those crucial genes to sleep, increasing the chances of developing cancer and those other dread diseases.

While it is nearly impossible to avoid some of these toxins in our air and water, you can take control of some of them to minimize your exposure, including:

- Avoid drinking or eating from plastic cups, plates, or utensils or storing leftovers in plastics.

- Minimize or eliminate your use of pesticides and herbicides in your yard and garden.

- Eat organic foods as much as possible to minimize pesticide exposure and GMOs in the farming process.

- Use natural insect repellant and sunscreens.

- Buy clothing that is washable; avoid dry cleaning, which is a source of toxic chemicals.

- If you own a home built before 1980, have it checked for asbestos.

- If you have a pool or hot tub, use an ozone-based filtration system or natural purification such as salt water systems to avoid exposure to toxic chlorine or bromine.

- Toss out toxic household cleaners and personal care products that contain known carcinogens.

These suggestions are just the tip of the iceberg. I could write a whole book on this subject. I won't do that though, since there are numerous excellent books on natural ways to survive and thrive in a toxic world.

Exercise is one last element of epigenetics. Don't take it lightly! There are several studies that prove that regular exercise keeps genes functioning as they are meant to function to prevent cancer.

MicroRNAs–the new frontier

One of the most exciting new discoveries in epigenetics and cancer is the identification of small genes, called microRNAs. You may remember from your high school biology classes that RNA carries genetic information.

MicroRNA, which I call miRNA, is a tiny amalgamation of molecules carrying a tiny bit of extremely powerful information.

I think of miRNAs as the high-ranking officers in the genetic army. Genes are simply privates in that army, the foot soldiers. We've only just discovered that miRNAs are the

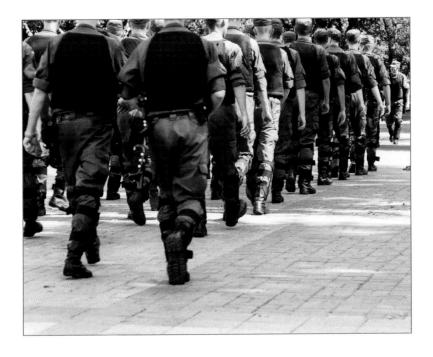

bosses, at least a colonel in the genetic army, that tells all the genes what to do. The "foot soldiers" obey without question.

This discovery means a compound that speaks directly to the miRNA has a profound effect all the way down the genetic "chain of command." A single miRNA molecule can control hundreds, maybe thousands of genes. It's much more efficient and potentially much more effective in maintaining perfect gene function that can otherwise govern your body's response to cancer triggers.

Think of it this way: If one colonel could blow the bugle and wake up 500 or 1,000 genes all at once, wouldn't that be preferable to trying to shake each soldier awake individually?

Pharmaceutical companies are now trying to develop drugs that will target miRNAs, designer drugs to hit the big bosses and the foot soldiers at the same time. Those designer drugs still lack the finesse we find in the wide variety of healing compounds that work synergistically in curcumin.

Curcumin is the colonel here. This powerful natural medicine can hit large numbers of genes all at once. My research team is probably one of the first to work on natural products, including curcumin, examining the mechanisms by which they influence the activity of miRNAs.

Part of the beauty of miRNAs is that targeting hundreds of genes is not a random process. There are very specific genes that activate or deactivate the cancer process, apoptosis and angiogenesis, as we'll discuss later. There are unique miRNAs for breast cancer, prostate cancer and colon cancer—all types of cancers. What if we could just have a persuasive conversation with the colonel of breast cancer, for example, and then leave the rest alone if they are functioning correctly? That's precisely what curcumin does. This is scientifically beautiful. It's uncanny and it's awe-inspiring.

In another decade, we may find the general who is in charge of the whole army, SuperRNA, but for now, I'm happy to be working with the colonels.

New cancer drugs and why they cause more problems than they solve

The pharmaceutical industry is hard at work looking for new cancer drugs based on epigenetics. It's not doing very well for a few fundamental reasons that they don't seem to comprehend.

Here's the problem: The newer drugs take a shotgun approach and completely turn on or turn off specific genes. Now, there are some genes that are turned off when we are born, to protect us. The genes that tell tumors to grow should stay turned off. We want them to stay asleep. But these "shotgun" drugs wake up everybody, so cancer growth in one part of the body might be slowed while it might be unintentionally sped up in other parts of the body.

If these shotgun approaches completely turn off an overactive gene, , this will force other genes and pathways to go haywire as they compensate for the loss of function of the gene that has been turned off by this drug. It's kind of like when you have an ancient plumbing system in your house and you replace only one of the pipes. It won't solve the problem. The new pipe may work just fine, but the old faulty system will result in leaks in other parts of the house.

Pharmaceutical drugs separate out one or two of the compounds found naturally in plants. They are built with a narrow target in mind. The drug has no way of controlling its activity, much like antibiotics that kill all bacteria in their path, taking out the good as well as the bad.

Plants, especially curcumin, have a built-in wisdom that awakens the genes that fight cancer and keeps the cancer-causing ones asleep. Curcumin is one of the natural plant compounds that offers a selective way of only waking up the genes that are supposed to be awake without alerting the bad guys. It restores the natural balance.

The evidence

The research on epigenetics is new and exciting. As of this writing, a search of the term "epigenetics" on the National Library of Medicine's database returns 11,514 results and "epigenetics and cancer" returns 4,375 studies—most of them in the past 15 years.

Here's some of the most important information we have from this research:

- Inherited gene mutations are rarely responsible for cancer. However, epigenetic alterations in genes are found in virtually all cancerous tumors.

- Cancer is a preventable disease through proper lifestyle, most often through a correct diet.

- Epigenetic changes can be reversed.

- Plant-based diets are powerful epigenetic cancer-prevention tools and can put the brakes on cancer-causing genes while waking up the cancer-preventing genes.

- Certain cancer-preventing genes sometimes go to sleep while other genes that are normally asleep in most humans can wake up and cause cancer.

Numerous fruits, vegetables, and herbs have proven to be helpful in creating epigenetic balance.

Curcumin and epigenetics

Your choice to eat organic fruits, vegetables and herbs in abundance is part of a smart plan to prevent and reverse cancer. But curcumin surpasses them all. Think of the epigenetic power of curcumin as your insurance policy, not only against cancer, but also against the other diseases I've mentioned in this chapter.

My own research has uncovered some truly exciting actions of curcumin for cancer prevention and for the treatment of several types of existing cancers.

- As a powerful antioxidant, it keeps cells reproducing exact copies of themselves, preventing the cellular damage and mutations that can lead to cancer and other degenerative diseases.

- It induces apoptosis, that genetic Grim Reaper that tells cells when it is their natural time to die instead of reproducing out of control and forming cancerous tumors.

- It turns on tumor-suppressing genes and turns off tumor-causing genes.

Finally

The majority of cancers are preventable. Clearly, an ounce of prevention is worth a pound of cure. Cancer prevention is preferable to treating an existing disease. There is ample scientific evidence that curcumin works both in prevention and in treatment.

Each day is a new day. If your lifestyle has not been optimal, you can change it today. The results will be a dramatically minimized risk of all types of cancer and a much more positive outlook if you have been diagnosed with cancer.

WHAT YOU NEED TO KNOW

◆ Only a small percentage of cancers are caused by "bad" genes. Most are caused by lifestyle choices, sometimes inherited from our families or our cultures. Epigenetics means that we can control our genes and their ability to fight cancer.

◆ Diet is the major element in turning on the cancer-preventing genes and turning off the cancer-causing genes.

◆ Minimizing your toxic exposure and committing to a regular exercise program will also keep genes functioning to prevent cancer.

◆ Curcumin contains the most powerful epigenetic compounds known to science. It helps turn on the sleeping cancer-preventing genes and turn off the cancer-causing ones that should be asleep.

◆ All chronic diseases, including cancer, diabetes and Alzheimer's, have an element of epigenetics and can be reversed through lifestyle changes. Changing the expression of these genes will help prevent these diseases, and will slow down the progression in people who are already ill. In some types of diseases, it may even be curative.

◆ In short, if I had any type of cancer or anyone in my family was in that position, I would absolutely use curcumin at all stages of the disease. I use it now and provide it for all my loved ones because prevention is always the best path.

How Cancer Starts, Stays and Spreads

Cancer cells are also unbelievably smart—smarter than your average healthy cells—and they will fight with a fury to survive.

Let's start with some simple terms that are important to moving forward with our understanding of cancer and how it starts, gains hold and spreads. We'll give you more details later in this chapter.

Apoptosis: Every single one of the trillions of cells in your body has a finite, or limited, lifespan. They are born, perform the tasks they are meant to perform, they reproduce and they die. This growth cycle of cells is a natural process called *apoptosis* or programmed cell death. There are genes that govern this natural process of cell death. Sometimes genes go into a deep slumber or become defective and stop doing their job. Then cells continue to live and reproduce long beyond their time, creating cancerous tumors.

In cancer cells, the genes that tell the cells to die go to sleep, which allows cancer cells to evade death. As the productive process goes on, more and more cells pile up, eventually becoming a large mass of cells known as tumors. There are also cancers that do not form solid masses, such as leukemia and lymphoma, but these malignancies are also a result of uncontrolled cells that are no longer instructed by their genes to die after reproduction.

Angiogenesis: This is the process by which these tumors create their own blood supply, which gives them nutrients and oxygen so they can thrive and grow. These cancers, driven by their hunger for survival, find ways to obtain what they need by creating their own system of blood vessels designed specifically to deliver nutrients and oxygen. This process, called *angiogenesis*, helps ensure the survival of the cancer cells and the disease.

Metastasis: Finally, cancers want to hedge their bets. Not only are those cells capable of feeding themselves, they are also capable of entering the bloodstream and spreading far and wide in the human body, the process called *metastasis.*

This is the spread of cancer from its origin, known as the primary site, to another part of the body. Part of cancer's innate mission to survive is for it to thrive.

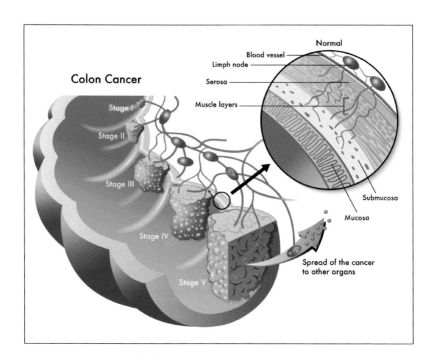

Anyone who has had cancer or loves someone with the disease dreads the news that the disease has spread. While not a death sentence in itself, metastasis signals the need to bring out all of the heavy artillery to fight the war on a second or even third front.

Now let's go into each of these three major terms individually and see how we can use epigenetics, and specifically, how we can use curcumin to prevent and even reverse these key elements of cancer.

Apoptosis: Cells that refuse to die

The formal explanation for apoptosis is programmed cell death. Every one of the 70 trillion cells in the human body, give or take a few, has a specific life span. Each cell is born an exact replica of its parent cell. It matures, reproduces creating offspring that are exact replicas of itself, and if it is working correctly, eventually it dies.

When the cell dies, the body releases specific proteins that break down the cell walls and the RNA (ribonucleic acid—genetic material) from the old cell, which shrinks and sends out a signal to the body's vacuum cleaner, called macrophages, to seamlessly eliminate it, leaving no trace.

Sometimes things go wrong. The instruction manual inside the cell gets damaged and the instructions for apoptosis are blotted out. There are too many living cells. The old cells that refuse to die become nearly immortal. In addition, old cells may have impaired genetic programming, so when they do reproduce, they may not make identical copies of themselves as nature intended. Old cells and young newly-formed cells are reproducing wildly and pile up. Instead of being flushed out of the system as happens naturally when cells die, these impaired and hyperactive cells form tumors, individually or in partnership with each other.

Remember, cancer cells are smart in their own way. They have figured out a way to make themselves immortal and to resist the body's chemical death signals. They also can themselves trigger complicated gene changes to escape apoptosis.

Some of these cancer cells are even resistant to conventional medicine's efforts to kill them. There are drugs that are geared toward causing those nearly immortal cells to die, but like most pharmaceuticals in the cancer industry, these drugs not only kill the cancer cells, but kill the normal cells as well, which is one of the reasons for the toxicity and side effects patients experience when they undergo chemotherapy.

How curcumin stops cancer cells that refuse to die

Remember the chapter on epigenetics and how curcumin wakes up sleeping genes and puts cancer-promoting genes to sleep? Well, there is also a genetic malfunction taking place when cells either refuse to die or are genetically triggered to reproduce wildly and uncontrollably.

Curcumin has a unique way of telling those apoptosis-inducing genes to wake up and end the lives of those death defying cancer cells or tell those wildly partying apoptosis-suppressing genes to return to their natural sleep state and stop forming tumors.

Curcumin selectively kills the cells that have outlived their lifespans without harming normal tissues. It reprograms the deficient genes to re-establish the natural life cycle of the cells. MiRNAs (remember those colonels that can command large numbers of cells?) come back into the picture here because they control large groups of genes and order them to do as they are told.

All of curcumin's healing power takes place without side effects, unlike the pharmaceutical drugs that can have serious and sometimes life-threatening side effects, killing cells needed for brain function or lung function or any of a million different body needs.

Curcumin works powerfully to eliminate those immortal cells. A secondary and longer-term process is to retrain the genes to stay awake and continue to perform their correct function so cancer does not return. This is one reason why most cancer patients should consider taking curcumin indefinitely, even years after they have been declared cancer free.

Keep taking curcumin, even if you are cancer free. This natural medicine will thwart the return of cancer.

Angiogenesis: Fierce survivalists

The term comes from the two Greek words *angio,* meaning blood vessel, and *genesis,* meaning beginning. In a positive sense, angiogenesis is a crucial part of the development of a baby in the womb as it grows, creating a circulatory system to support critical organs like bones, skin and brain. Angiogenesis continues throughout our lives, usually for good purposes, like healing wounds or repairing damage.

It's part of a delicate balance between normal and healthy blood vessel growth intended to keep the body nourished and the destructive network of capillaries that feed malignant tumors.

Those tumors begin with abnormal clumpings of cells that didn't get the messages that it was time to die. Now they have become expert survivalists.

In their urgent quest to survive, the tumor cells release specific sets of chemical signals that command the body to produce a network of blood vessels that will feed the tumor, provide it with nutrients and oxygen, ensuring its ability to grow, thrive, and survive. These selfish cancer cells then are able to shuttle nutrition and oxygen from healthy cells to feed themselves.

Once a tumor has established its own blood vessel network, it becomes immeasurably stronger. It can easily send signals for further development of enhanced circulation to feed even more and larger tumors. Treatment becomes far more difficult.

What we want to do is induce tumor "hypoxia"—to literally starve the tumor by cutting off its oxygen and nutrient supply.

Some types of cancer therapy target these abnormal blood vessels, working on the theory that cancerous tumors cannot grow beyond about the size of a pinhead without a blood supply.

These recently-developed therapies include a relatively new class of drugs called angiogenesis inhibitors that are intended to starve tumors to death. They work—for a small percentage of patients—by blocking the signals sent by those brilliant cancer cells calling for blood supply.

The handful of drugs designated for this purpose have serious side effects, as do most chemotherapy drugs, including increased high blood pressure, risk of stroke or heart attack, gastrointestinal perforations (that is a rupture of the stomach or intestine), slow wound healing, severe bleeding and birth defects.

How curcumin works to stop angiogenesis

Researchers from Emory University concluded in a 2007 study that curcumin has "enormous potential" to stop angiogenesis. They found that curcumin interrupted the cell signals sent by malignant cells calling for the formation of new blood vessels.

Lab studies show curcumin is particularly effective in preventing the formation of a blood supply to melanoma cells, effectively stopping one of the most virulent and deadly forms of skin cancer.

It tells genes not to activate VEGF (vascular endothelial growth factor) that triggers the formation of new blood vessel networks to feed tumors.

Curcumin also stops the tumor's ability to steal nutrients from healthy cells.

Metastasis: Alien invaders

Metastasis is the spread of cancer from a primary site to another. It's the third leg of the stool that explains how cancer starts, gets a foothold and kills.

Here's what happens and how it's connected to apoptosis and angiogenesis:

Those immortal cells (the result of a deficiency in the natural process of apoptosis) have clumped together to form tumors. Then they have developed their own food supply (angiogenesis) and finally, they find a way to spread themselves throughout the body (metastasis) to ensure their survival.

There is a second stage of angiogenesis, called lymph angiogenesis, in which the blood vessels surrounding the tumor begin to migrate into the lymphatic system. (You may

Metastasis: How Cancer Spreads

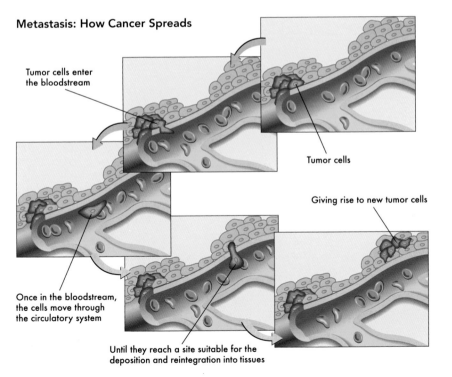

Tumor cells enter the bloodstream

Tumor cells

Giving rise to new tumor cells

Once in the bloodstream, the cells move through the circulatory system

Until they reach a site suitable for the deposition and reintegration into tissues

recall from your high school biology that the lymph system is a vast network of vessels and a vital part of the immune system that constantly sweeps bacteria and other pathogens out of the body.)

The cancer cells are able to travel through the lymphatic system, eventually winding up in lymph nodes. From there it's an easy trip from the lymphatic system to the bloodstream, and then they can go wherever they want. That explains how cancer can spread to distant organs, for example from the ovaries to the lung or from the breast to the bones.

In short, angiogenesis insures the survival of the cancer cells in the short-term. Metastasis promotes long-term survival of the cancer and gives it the opportunity to invade many organs.

Of course, these metastases are what will eventually kill the human body, and in the process, will also kill the tumors, but they really aren't all that smart or that predictive to recognize that their strategy winds up being fatal for both the host and the cancer.

How curcumin works to stop metastasis

A review conducted by Singaporean researchers took an in-depth look at 315 studies on curcumin and its effectiveness against a wide variety of cancers at all stages. Their comments on the "multifaceted" ways curcumin prevents and treats cancer are quite exciting:

"Despite significant advances in treatment modalities over the last decade, neither the incidence of the disease nor the mortality due to cancer has altered in the last thirty years. Available anticancer drugs exhibit limited efficacy, associated with severe side effects and are also expensive. Thus, identification of pharmacological agents that do not have these disadvantages is required. Curcumin, a polyphenolic compound derived from turmeric (*curcumin longa*), is one such agent that has been extensively studied over the last three to four decades for its potential anti-inflammatory and/or anticancer effects. *Curcumin has been found to suppress initiation, progression and metastasis of a variety of tumors."*

This particular study carefully examined the results of these hundreds of previous studies confirming curcumin's effectiveness against a wide variety of cancers, including:

- Cancerous lesions

- Lung cancer

- Colorectal cancer

- Liver metastases from colorectal cancer

- Multiple myeloma

- Advanced pancreatic cancer

- Advanced and metastatic breast cancer

- Prostate cancer

- Head and neck cancer

- Chronic myeloid leukemia

All of these types of cancer are well known to metastasize aggressively, which is why they are among the most fatal types of cancers.

It's easy to see from this narrative how powerful curcumin is against cancer and the numerous ways it attacks the origination, growth and spread of cancer.

WHAT YOU NEED TO KNOW

So we have a spiral here—or a vicious circle, if you like:

- *Apoptosis* allows cells to live beyond their natural lifespan.

- *Angiogenesis* creates life-giving nutrient networks to feed those bundles of cancer cells and allows them to grow.

- *Metastasis,* creating new tumors in other parts of the body, which build up more masses of cancer cells, and new nutrient networks, and new metastases that will eventually kill the host human if the cycle is not broken.

Hundreds of recent studies confirm curcumin's abilities to interrupt these deadly activities at a wide variety of entry points, working as a "multifaceted" approach to cancer at all stages.

CHAPTER 6

Stop Cancer from Returning

By reading this far, you've probably come to some of the same conclusions I have.

First is that we must all recognize that cancer cells are the geniuses of the biochemical world. They're undoubtedly smarter than your average brain, bone or skin cell. Cancer cells are driven by self-preservation, with strength far beyond the survival instincts of normal cells. Like all life forms, they fight like demons to survive, but they are also incredibly intelligent, enough to thwart most attempts to kill them. It's almost like they have their own brains.

You'll note I said, "most," but not "all" attempts to kill them. Curcumin steps in to interrupt the best-laid plans of genius cancer cells.

Here are three new areas for us to examine:

- Cancer stem cells: Super cells that govern other cancer cells and are astonishingly difficult to kill.

- Chemo-resistance: Cancers that become resistant to chemo-therapeutic drugs that once worked.

- Chemo-sensitization: Making cancer cells more receptive to accepting the drugs that will eventually kill them.

Cancer stem cells

We've already established that most of us know someone who has had cancer. You probably already know that even with the standard cancer treatments—surgery, chemotherapy, and radiation, or any combination of these—cancer often returns. It may be three or four years or even longer, but those resistant cancer cells find a way to hide and survive, and some eventually emerge again and thrive. These are *cancer stem cells* and they can be deadly. When cancers return, they tend to be far more vicious and more aggressive than they were the first time around.

When a child is conceived, the egg and the sperm divide into a handful of healthy stem cells. Stem cells are the point of origination for all tissues in the body. Malleable like a child's

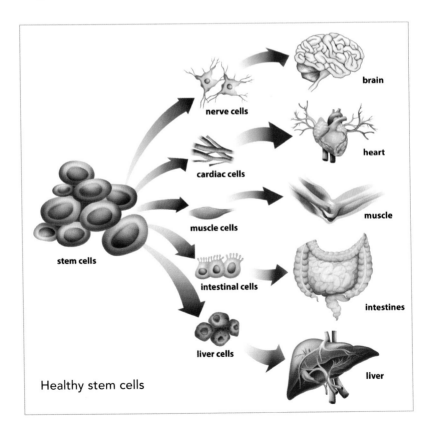

brain

nerve cells

heart

cardiac cells

muscle

muscle cells

intestinal cells

intestines

stem cells

liver cells

liver

Healthy stem cells

Play-Doh, stem cells can become any kind of cell. They can be brain cells, heart cells, pancreas cells, skin cells or hair and nail cells. Stem cells are the superheroes of the body, full of unlimited potential.

Cancer stem cells are different. We are not born with cancer stem cells. They are a tiny subset of cancer cells themselves. They are called this because they can be the point of origination for a cancer recurrence. They can disguise themselves and lie low, avoiding chemo and radiation therapy. Then when the coast is clear, they can spring forward and start making cancer cells again.

Cancer stem cells initiate and maintain cancer, and contribute to recurrence and drug resistance. Almost like the multi-tasking white-hatted miRNAs that combat cancer, these are their alter-egos, super-cells that govern other cancer cells and command them to grow and proliferate.

Cancer stem cells are immortal—or nearly so. As we've learned in earlier chapters, cancer cells do not have a normal lifespan like healthy cells. They live on and on, reproducing in their twisted fashion, creating more cancer cells and larger tumors that spread throughout the body.

In addition, these cancer stem cells have an uncanny ability to hide from conventional medicine's diagnostic "radar," hiding in the deepest recesses of the body, appearing to sleep or staying quiet for months, even years, before they awaken and begin to grow again with a vengeance.

Researchers at the National Cancer Institute (NCI) suggested in a 2012 study that "inappropriate consumption of certain foods" might encourage cancer cell growth. Those same researchers also noted that curcumin has been scientifically proven to convince those unique master cells — cancer stem cells—to die at the right time.

This is a huge and exciting step forward in cancer treatment, buried in the usually dry and unemotional scientific jargon from the NCI. Curcumin may well be one of the most powerful substances known to science when it comes to eradicating cancer stem cells.

The same researchers note that even in particularly aggressive pancreatic and brain cancers, the "alarm clocks" or signaling pathways that wake up these cancer stem cells over time are shut down by curcumin. This humble botanical quite literally interrupts the chain of command between cancer stem cell colonels and the foot soldiers or ordinary cancer cells. When the colonels can no longer tell the foot soldiers what to do, they will eventually desert the cancer army, so they are no longer a threat.

My scientific community is in general agreement that targeting cancer stem cells is "a very promising concept and therapeutic option to eradicate tumors and prohibit resistance and recurrence."

Curcumin works in many ways. In particular, it disrupts the ability of the cancer stem cells to communicate with the ordinary cancer cells. Those cancer stem cells can morph into hundreds of different types of cells, all of them malignant.

In fact, University of Michigan research suggests that curcumin molecules are as smart as their malignant opponents because they can seek out cancer stem cells (breast cancer in that particular study) and attack them, but, unlike chemotherapy drugs, do not harm healthy stem cells or any other cells at all.

> Cancer stem cells can sometimes survive chemotherapy, and their survival is one of the main reasons why cancer can return after a few months or years in most patients.

Chemo-resistance

In all my years of cancer research, I have learned that almost every cancer patient develops some degree of resistance to chemotherapy drugs.

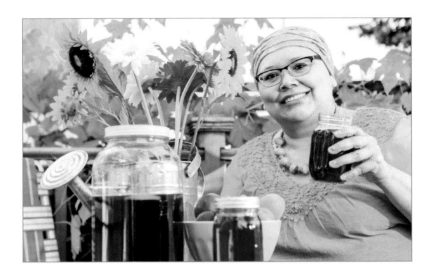

This means that chemotherapy drugs that were effective in the earlier phases of treatment almost always stop working over time. The tumors become resistant to the drug's intended effects and cancer cells continue to grow unchecked.

These cancer cells can be fooled once if they've never been exposed to a chemo drug before. The drug may destroy 95% or more of the cancer cells. The cells the chemo does not kill are the ones left to reproduce. The cancer becomes resistant to that drug. Regardless of what we throw at them, they figure out a way to develop resistance to one drug after another until we have nothing else to offer.

You already know that cancer cells have a hyper-survival mechanism. In simple terms, they don't want to die. Remember our examination of apoptosis, or programmed cell death in Chapter 5? Well, many chemo drugs target the apoptosis pathways, reminding those nearly immortal cancer cells when it's their time to die.

Over time, those genius cancer cells figure out a way to shut down the message. They overrule the command to bring back the natural pattern of cell death, allowing the cancer to continue to grow and spread.

Of course, they also are able to overcome the command to stop supplying nutrients to the cell clusters, overcoming all efforts to starve them.

Didn't I tell you these cancer cells are smart?

Cancer stem cells are even stronger and more resistant to conventional therapies than those foot soldier cancer cells.

So the patient has already undergone at least one course of chemotherapy, complete with myriad side effects that can include nausea, hair loss, weight loss, muscle wasting, extreme fatigue, organ damage and more, only to learn that the cancer has returned.

The only option most doctors can offer is another course of chemotherapy with a different drug, administered in the hope that the new drug will trick the genius cancer cells into committing suicide.

The vicious cycle has been set. Some of the cancer cells will die, but, until now, there have always been survivalist cancer cells that will hide out in the physiological wilderness and come back again another day.

Cancer very often returns, perhaps in the same place, perhaps in another part of the body. Doctors try another form of chemo. The patient weakens. Quality of life deteriorates to the point where it becomes intolerable. The outcome has been set almost from the beginning: The doctors eventually announce they can offer nothing else to overcome those cancer cells. The patient, in utter despair at the thought of more life-consuming drugs, loses hope.

It's a horrible story that too many of us have witnessed, if not experienced for ourselves. It's heartbreaking and it doesn't have to be this way at all.

What causes chemo-resistance? You've probably already got a good idea: Those cancer stem cells with their superpowers are able to escape, evolve and hide from all known chemotherapy drugs.

Curcumin's role

And how does curcumin fit into this picture? Curcumin:

- Sensitizes cancer cells—softens them up, if you will—so chemotherapy drugs can be more effective.

- Reminds cancer cells to die, to reinstate programmed cell death or apoptosis.

- Neutralizes the cells' over-developed survival mechanism.

- Finds alternate ways of carrying out the business of killing cancer cells, outpacing the rapid-fire "intelligence" of the cancer cells' abilities to resist new drug therapies.

Most of my work has been on colorectal cancer, but we know from numerous other studies that curcumin's value extends to many other types of cancer, perhaps encompassing all types of cancers.

My study in 2013 was unique because we created a colon cancer laboratory model that mimicked the human situation. We started treating colon cancer cells with different types of chemotherapy at different dosages until the cells became unresponsive to the drugs and stopped dying. Eventually, even when treated with 10 times, 50 times and even 100 times higher dosages of the chemo drugs, the cells refused to die. Interestingly, nothing killed these incredibly tough cancer cells until we brought in curcumin.

The curcumin activated everything that was needed to eliminate the cancer stem cells: angiogenesis, apoptosis and epigenetics. The cells died. This was tremendously exciting!

Then we injected those chemo-resistant cancer cells into animals and we found the same effect. We're now planning similar research with advanced stage multi-drug resistant colon cancer patients. People with end stage colon cancer cannot expect to survive more than a few months. If we can give them curcumin, we may well be able to extend their lives by a month or two, or even six months, with a vastly improved quality of life. It may not be a cure, but it can certainly make a positive difference.

Chemo-sensitization

This is a glass half full/glass half empty topic. Chemo-sensitivity or chemo-enhancement is the opposite of chemo-resistance. It means that curcumin has been found to actually help sensitize cancer cells, specifically those notoriously tough cancer stem cells, making them vulnerable to destruction by chemotherapy drugs, ending their resistance and allowing them to be killed by the drugs.

One of our studies confirms that curcumin helped improve the effectiveness of 5-fluorouracil (5-FU), a chemotherapy drug often used in patients with colorectal cancer. Although this study has been published, our research is ongoing. Our theory is that curcumin helps activate those miRNA colonels to overcome chemo-resistant cancer stem cells providing for far more effective treatment.

There is other research that confirms our theory and expands upon it, showing that curcumin increases sensitivity to several types of chemotherapy drugs in a variety of cancers: breast, colon, pancreas, gastric, liver, blood, lung, prostate, bladder, cervix, ovary, head and neck. By making the cancer cells more vulnerable to chemotherapy drugs, we have a vastly improved chance of defeating the cancers with lower doses of toxic drugs and less harm to the patient.

This includes advanced cancers that are considered inoperable.

In addition to 5-FU, research has confirmed that curcumin enhances the effectiveness of several other drugs used to treat advanced colon cancers, including irinotecan, FOLFOX, gemcitabine and celecoxib.

There's another exciting addition in the chemo-sensitivity arena: We've found that curcumin also increases the effectiveness of radiation therapy *and* it helps protect important organs like the liver, kidneys, oral mucosa and heart from the toxic side effects of chemotherapy and radiation.

Curcumin is a safe and effective choice
during every stage of cancer, on its own or when
combined with chemo or radiation therapy.

Finally

Curcumin has uncanny healing and preventive powers. It does everything possible to counteract the destructive powers of cancer stem cells. My research shows that curcumin eliminates significantly more cancer stem cells than any other natural therapy currently known.

Will curcumin eliminate the cancer stem cells forever? Maybe yes, maybe no. We have studied this aspect of curcumin for several years and, while we need more research, I feel quite optimistic that ongoing and future studies of curcumin in humans will show us that curcumin can provide a cure or a much, much longer remission time than we now know.

In short, if I had any type of cancer or anyone in my family was in that position, I would absolutely use curcumin at all stages of the disease.

Most likely it would stop the disease from progressing. There are no serious side effects (sometimes a bit of loose stools at very high doses).

Of course, ideally, we can all use curcumin for prevention along with other healthy lifestyle habits and the cancer never gets a foothold. But if you or someone you love does get any type of cancer, you definitely should talk to your oncologist about using curcumin. Why not? There is nothing to lose and everything to gain.

WHAT YOU NEED TO KNOW

◆ **Stem cells:** We're adding a new component to the vicious cycle of cancer. These cells have a super-enhanced will to live and are able to overcome almost all efforts to kill them known to conventional medicine. Their ability to escape detection is the primary reason why most cancers recur after conventional treatment.

◆ **Chemo-resistance:** Cancer cells, and particularly cancer stem cells, are able to become resistant to chemotherapy drugs in only a few generations, so chemotherapy no longer works after a period of time. Eventually, doctors run out of options.

◆ **Chemo-enhancement:** This is the other aspect of curcumin's ability to overcome chemo-resistance, so when given with some conventional chemotherapy drugs, research shows that it can actually make the chemo drugs work better.

Curcumin's ability to overcome the superpowers of cancer stem cells, eliminating chemo-resistance and enhancing the effectiveness of chemotherapy drugs is unparalleled, without any of the terrible side effects that almost always accompany conventional cancer treatment.

CHAPTER 7

Curcumin as an Integrative Therapy

So—you or someone you love has been diagnosed with cancer.

Your brain is whirling. You are unable to assimilate anything. You have a million questions, but you're unable to voice any of them.

That's the first step-the day you get the news. The C-word. It's devastating.

Next you ask, "Why me?" "Why my husband, my mother, my child?"

Then in a nanosecond, your friends rush in to "help." Many of them have cancer stories to tell you—each one more dire than the last. Others want you to take coffee enemas, go to a clinic in Mexico, or adopt a macrobiotic diet. Everyone has a wonder "cure."

Your confusion grows.

Your doctors want to do chemotherapy and radiation, possibly surgery. You've seen the devastating effects of all of these, but you are terrified that you'll make the wrong choice, the fatal choice.

Doctors disparage "alternative" therapies as quackery. Friends and alternative practitioners urge you to try herbs, machines, and avoid chemo and radiation at all costs.

You are facing a potentially life-threatening illness; you're frightened and overwhelmed, overloaded with "information," with no tools to determine what's true and what's not. You have no idea where to turn.

Ask, "Is it really cancer?"

In recent years, we have seen vastly increased numbers of cancer diagnoses. With the advances in technology, we now have the ability to diagnose cancers much earlier. We also can find cells that may be precancerous or look abnormal. Yes, we have better diagnostic tools. But that doesn't necessarily mean we need to engage in aggressive cancer treatment when there are abnormal cells that may or may not even be cancer. In many cases, the treatment (surgery, chemotherapy and radiation have become standard for most types of cancer) is far more destructive to the human body than the cancer itself would ever be.

Most of us by now have heard of men diagnosed with prostate cancers that are so slow growing that doctors are telling men in their 60s or older that something else will kill them before cancer ever does. That's a somewhat new and enlightened position for conventional medicine, but it's only a drop in the bucket.

But here's the point: Most of us may have some type of abnormal cells if we look carefully enough. Does this mean we all have cancer? Of course not! However, the discovery of any abnormal cells may actually be a red flag, an impetus that we need to make the lifestyle changes that will keep these cells from becoming a disease.

This notion brings into focus all of the epigenetic and lifestyle changes that cause gene disruptions that can lead to cancer.

Look to science

If you've been diagnosed with cancer and you're not satisfied with the answers from your doctor, you probably won't be surprised that I recommend you look at the science behind the recommendation, both on the "alternative" side and the conventional medical treatment side.

I don't really like to call it "alternative." That's old terminology. Today, natural therapies are more often called complementary or integrative therapies. That makes sense to me.

I would like to offer you another way of thinking about a cancer diagnosis: If you choose, you can effectively combine natural remedies and conventional treatment.

In the past 20 years, dietary supplements have become part of the Western culture. More than half of the U.S. population regularly uses dietary supplements. Supplement and herbal remedy sales alone in 2010 totaled $5.2 billion, according to a 2013 study published in the journal, *Integrative Cancer Therapies*.

Cancer patients are particularly likely to use supplements, with as many as 87% of breast cancer patients using some type of dietary supplement. In the late '90s, about 20% of cancer patients used some kind of supplements designed to slow their cancers. Today, that figure is closer to 60%. Why? Because they've seen the benefits when family members and friends have used them *and* there is science behind many of them.

Doctors say "No"

It's interesting to note that many cancer patients do not report their supplement use to their doctors, perhaps for fear of being ridiculed or encountering negativity. Some doctors reflexively say "no" to complementary therapies when their patients ask about them, often a result of ignorance about the broad scope of scientific evidence that supports their value.

Many doctors will tell you that these supplements have no scientific validation. I'm here to tell you that in many instances that may not be true and may simply be a smokescreen for the doctor's lack of knowledge.

I don't intend to categorize the medical profession here. But you are very likely to find that many doctors subscribe to a pretty rigid way of thinking about what works and what doesn't work.

A good doctor will do some research on supplements that a patient wants to use and endorse the ones that have scientific validation and discourage the use of those that might be ineffective or even harmful. I strongly believe that a relationship of trust between a physician and a patient is an essential part of the healing process.

For example, a search of the National Library of Medicine's database of published scientific studies on curcumin returns 8,237 results as of this writing and adding cancer to the search, you'll find 3,121 results, the earliest in 1983.

This is a substantial body of science that proves curcumin's power, much of it as a cancer preventive and treatment. I know. I've conducted several of those studies myself.

There is undeniable evidence that curcumin should be one of our most valuable weapons in our arsenal against cancer. It may even be the most effective one. You can take that information to your doctor with confidence.

You'll note that I have included a brief synopsis of the key scientific points on this topic in Chapter 13. I encourage you to copy those pages and give them to your doctor. While doctors may not have time to read an entire book, please impress upon your medical professionals the importance of reading and assimilating these few key pages. It could quite literally save your life and the lives of many others.

Chemo-enhancement

Some of the best research shows that curcumin can increase the effectiveness of chemotherapy drugs and radiation therapy. Plus, curcumin can protect surrounding tissues from the damage frequently caused by chemo drugs.

Let me give you just a few important examples:

In my own research on colorectal cancer, in six published studies, we definitively proved that the combination of curcumin with 5-FU (5-fluorouracil) *is far more effective in reducing the size of tumors and making them more sensitive to the drug than either curcumin or the drug alone.*

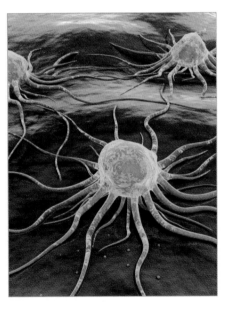

Researchers at MD Anderson Cancer Center combined curcumin and gemcitabine, a chemotherapy drug used to treat pancreatic cancer, one of the most aggressive and most frequently fatal cancers. In their research published in 2010, they found that curcumin and gemcitabine used together were a powerful team. The combination therapy increased programmed cell death (apoptosis) in those cancer cells and prevented them from developing their own nutrient supplies (angiogenesis). Perhaps even more significantly, curcumin helped the chemo drug to be more effective for a longer period of time, overcoming the chemo-resistance that almost always emerges.

Finally, there are several studies that show curcumin enhances the effectiveness of paclitaxel, a chemotherapy agent used to treat breast cancer. In my own research, published in 2010, we reviewed the effectiveness of curcumin in enhancing several different chemotherapy drugs and radiation therapy while protecting healthy tissues.

Research on a wide variety of chemotherapy agents used to treat a wide variety of cancers confirms the synergistic effect when curcumin is added to the treatment regimen. These types of cancer include:

- Prostate
- Multiple myeloma
- Ovarian
- Leukemia
- Gastric
- Liver
- Cervical
- Breast
- Pancreatic
- Lung
- Bladder
- Brain
- Many more . . .

Other research confirms the usefulness of combining curcumin with radiation therapy, especially in treating difficult brain, head and neck cancers.

By now, you're surely beginning to see curcumin's ability to attack cancer from a number of angles. Without any question, curcumin surpasses any other natural or synthetic substance in its approach to cancer. It's exciting!

As a scientist, I'm very cautious about being overly exuberant, but it's impossible to overstate the promise of curcumin in preventing and treating, perhaps even curing, cancer. This is integrative medicine at its best.

A potent herbal combo

I have to mention here another synergistic effect, the combination of curcumin and another herb, called boswellia. This is one combination with which I am very familiar since my study on the combined effects of these two herbs was published in 2015 in the journal, *Cancer Prevention Research*. We found that curcumin and boswellic acid, from the *Boswellia serrata* plant commonly known as frankincense, worked together through the miRNA genes to reduce inflammation, suppress tumor growth, reduce the size of existing tumors, initiate pro-grammed cell death (apoptosis) in laboratory analyses of col-orectal cell lines and in animals with colorectal cancer at a much greater rate than either herb alone would achieve.

The curcumin-boswellia combination actually reduced tumor growth in laboratory animals within as little as two days of treatment! It also increased the responsiveness to treatment in people with the p53 gene mutation that occurs in about half of colorectal cancer patients.

As always, the formulations of these herbs are important for maximum availability to our bodies. My research on cur-cumin used the BCM-95™ formulation, a non-toxic extraction method that science shows us has enhanced absorption and contains turmerones from turmeric essential oils not found in other curcumin formulations. This form also includes turmeric essential oil, which itself has anticancer properties as well. health properties.

The boswellia extraction I have studied called Bospure™ is standardized to contain higher levels of AKBA (acetyl-keto-beta-boswellic acid, the active ingredient in boswellia) and purified to remove virtually all beta-boswellic acid, a com-pound that causes inflammation. This results in better anti-inflammatory effects.

Clearly, there is an abundance of scientific research that confirms not only the effectiveness of curcumin as a standalone against cancer, but shows its ability to magnify the effects of standard cancer therapies. If you have been diagnosed with any type of cancer, I urge you to urge you doctor to investigate the value of curcumin with no negative side effects.

WHAT YOU NEED TO KNOW

- Curcumin is at the top of most lists of supplements that have powerful anticancer effects.

- Curcumin is a valid choice for treatment of a variety of types of cancer.

- Curcumin is scientifically validated to enhance the effectiveness of conventional cancer treatments, including chemotherapy and radiation while protecting healthy cells from the damage associated with cancer treatments.

- In combination with boswellia, curcumin can have a synergistic effect both in preventing and treating cancer.

PART 2

Curcumin and Other Chronic Inflammatory Diseases

CHAPTER 8

Depression, Alzheimer's and Dementia

B rain health is at the core of who we are as humans. If you have a healthy brain, you have an inquiring mind, you are engaged in the world around you, you communicate clearly with others and form nurturing relationships. You remember what you need to remember, and you have good judgment.

There are sometimes emotionally painful alterations in the ability of our bodies to manufacture or balance brain chemicals (also called neurotransmitters) that govern a wide array of brain functions. This can result in depression. Brain chemistry malfunctions also occur when brain cells begin to die, abnormal proteins start to accumulate, and the brain starts to shrink, resulting in memory loss and Alzheimer's disease, the most common form of dementia.

Curcumin's unique ability to cross the blood-brain barrier means that it can affect brain chemistry and the survival mechanisms of brain cells (neurons). It has preventive and healing effects that few other nutrients can offer.

Imbalances in neurotransmitters, the brain chemicals that are the computer that controls virtually every function of the human body, play a role in depression, Alzheimer's disease, other forms of dementia, and many other brain disorders.

Let's look at depression and Alzheimer's disease (AD) separately, since they are very different diseases. However, it has been recently demonstrated that people who suffer with depression have a higher risk of AD than the general population, so there are certain commonalities that apply to both diseases.

Depression

Depressive disorder is a crushing inability to cope with life and the world.

Over a lifetime, 16.5% of the U.S. adult population (18.8 million people) suffers from a major depressive disorder and 30% of those cases are so severe that depression impairs the ability to work or even to function in the world in normal terms.

We know that women are 70% more likely to develop depression than men, that Caucasians have a 40% higher risk for depression than African-Americans and that people between the ages of 18 and 29 are at much greater risk of major depression than people over 60.

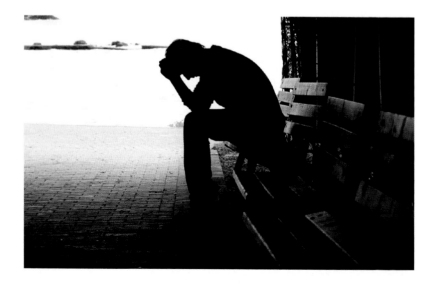

Depression affects children as well. Government statistics show 4.7% of 13- to 18-year olds suffer from severe mood disorders and girls are nearly twice as vulnerable as boys. The rate of teen depression is increasing by an alarming 23% per year.

We're not talking about the occasional day or even days of feeling blue. We're not talking about the normal ups and downs of life, the loss of a relationship, the loss of a job or even the loss of a loved one. Depression is not sadness.

Depressive disorder is a crushing inability to cope with life and the world. It creates apathy, hopelessness, fatigue, sleep disorders and even physical pain. Yet only about half of its sufferers get treatment and 80% of the treatment is completely ineffective.

Standard medical treatment for depression is usually a series of antidepressant pharmaceuticals with a high risk of serious side effects and low rates of effectiveness. Research shows that antidepressants work for only 35 to 45% of the population and some figures suggest the response rate is as low as 30%. Worse yet, antidepressants like Prozac, Paxil and Zoloft have been linked to suicide, violence, psychosis, abnormal bleeding and brain tumors.

What causes depression? Certainly short-term depression can be the result of life events, as can long-term trauma, such as sexual abuse and a family history of depression.

Most people with depression have high levels of inflammation in the brain and a decreased ability to create new brain cells, a process called "neurogenesis." They become deficient in mood-lifting serotonin, motivating noradrenaline and sleep-enhancing tryptophan because the brain is not working correctly.

Curcumin offers solutions to brain chemistry imbalances. It relieves inflammation and stimulates the formation of new brain cells through neurogenesis. This results in a better balance of neurotransmitters. Curcumin enhances noradrenaline and tryptophan levels and increases the production of dopamine, another neurotransmitter that controls emotional response and the ability to experience pleasure and pain.

Numerous studies underscore curcumin's ability to improve levels of neurotransmitters and thereby improve mood.

Curcumin not only manages the symptoms of depression, it goes much deeper by treating the underlying causes.

Many people accidentally stumble on curcumin's antidepressant action when they take it for another condition, most typically to address joint pain. The action is so subtle that some users have written that they didn't realize their depression had disappeared until they stopped taking curcumin and the depression returned.

Because the effects of clinical depression are so variable, the severity of an individual's level of depression is often ranked by doctors on the Hamilton Depression Rating Scale. It includes questions about mood, feelings of guilt, suicide ideation, insomnia, anxiety, weight loss and more.

Scientific proof

We compared the effects of anti-depression drugs and curcumin in a study published in the journal, *Phytotherapy Research* in 2014. The study found the synergistic effects I had also noticed between curcumin and cancer chemotherapy drugs.

We selected 60 patients with major depressive disorder and randomly assigned them to one of the three groups:

- Fluoxetine (Prozac) 20 mg

- Curcumin BCM-95™ 500 mg twice daily

- Combination of fluoxetine and curcumin at the same dosage levels

Over a six-week period, people who got Prozac had a 64.7% improvement in their depression symptoms and a similar improvement—62.5%—for those who got curcumin only. That was significant enough in itself, since curcumin has no side effects and has similar effectiveness, while there are major side effects associated with the use of Prozac and other antidepressants, including anxiety, weight gain, digestive problems, erratic heart rate and more.

However, what we found next was the even more impressive: There is a synergistic effect between the two. Those who received both curcumin and fluoxetine had an impressively higher success rate: 77.8% improvement on the Hamilton scale.

There is a great deal more research on curcumin and depression. Here are some highlights:

Increases serotonin and dopamine levels: Several studies support curcumin's ability to boost mood by increasing levels of mood-enhancing neurotransmitters.

Acts like pharmaceutical drugs without the risks: Other research confirms that curcumin performs as well as other pharmaceutical antidepressants without the risks.

Antioxidant and anti-inflammatory mood improvement: Researchers are clearly enthusiastic about curcumin. Several studies further the body of evidence in favor of curcumin's positive effects on mood.

Alzheimer's disease and dementia

Dementia has often been called "The Long Goodbye," because it takes such a terrible toll on its victims and their families, usually for years until the inevitable end.

Alzheimer's is probably the best-known and most common form of dementia that gets worse over time and affects memory, thinking and behavior.

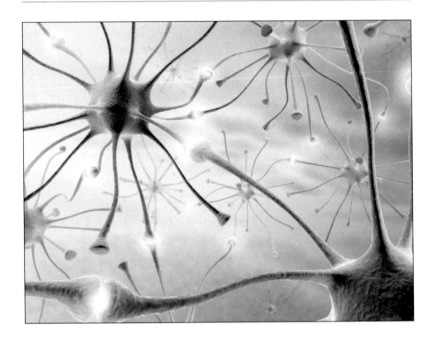

The National Institutes of Health estimates that more than 5 million Americans have Alzheimer's. Most of them are over 60, although there is an increasing rate of early onset Alzheimer's that can begin as early as the 30s.

Curcumin holds great promise for those with dementia and hope for people with Alzheimer's and their families.

There is a much lower rate of Alzheimer's disease in India, where curcumin and turmeric are part of a lifelong diet eaten several times a day. In fact, the rate of Alzheimer's in India among people ages 70–79 is about one quarter of the rate in the U.S. where curcumin and turmeric are rarely included in the standard diet.

Some of the most interesting research shows curcumin can:

Grow new brain cells: Until recently, scientists believed that it was impossible to grow new brain cells, but they dispelled that myth with the discovery of neurogenesis, the scientifically validated creation of new brain cells. University of Florida researchers have now confirmed that curcumin stimulates the birth of new neurons, particularly in the hippocampus, the seat of memory in the human brain.

Protect brain cells: Authors of a study published in the journal *Current Alzheimer's Research,* were enthusiastic about the antioxidant properties of curcumin to prevent brain cell deterioration and death. Inflammatory cells called cytokines have a role in speeding up Alzheimer's and the abilities of curcumin to inhibit the natural production of the anti-inflammatory COX-2 enzyme can help protect those brain cells.

Destroy plaques and tangles: Scientists at UCLA called curcumin "anti-amyloid" for its ability to overcome the beta-amyloid protein that forms the plaques and tangles characteristic of Alzheimer's. They also noted that people with Alzheimer's show signs of inflammation in their brains and credit curcumin's anti-inflammatory properties with an ability to address that problem. Another UCLA animal study showed curcumin supplements reduced substances believed to cause plaque by 43 to 45%. Some researchers have suggested curcumin binds directly to plaques and eliminates them.

Improve memory in people with Alzheimer's: An exciting Veteran's Administration study explores multiple ways in which curcumin not only prevents Alzheimer's and slows the progression of the disease, but actually improves memory in people already diagnosed with the disease.

Although doctors are highly unlikely to recommend curcumin for the treatment of these brain-related diseases, if I had a loved one suffering from one of them, I'd be very eager to give it to them.

What You Need to Know

◆ Curcumin's impressive anti-inflammatory effects make it a powerful tool in balancing brain chemistry and overcoming depression, Alzheimer's disease and dementia.

◆ Curcumin was shown in a human study to have a synergistic effect with the antidepressant pharmaceutical fluoxetine (Prozac™), offering a vastly improved option for success.

◆ Curcumin improves memory in people with Alzheimer's and attacks some of the basic symptoms of the disease and may offer reversal and even remission of the disease.

CHAPTER 9

Arthritis and Joint Pain

Virtually all of us experience occasional joint or back pain. With luck, it goes away with time, rest and perhaps an occasional ice pack. Sometimes it does not.

Each year, about 30 million of us visit a doctor complaining of joint pain. Another 40 million or so visit a doctor looking for relief from back pain. Add in 1.5 million people with rheumatoid arthritis, 6.1 million with gout, 5 million with fibromyalgia and 1.5 million broken bones suffered every year by people with osteoporosis and you'll see the magnitude of this painful problem.

Long-term musculoskeletal pain affects your entire being. It drains energy and contributes to chronic stress, a condition that has a myriad of negative side effects of its own, including obesity, metabolic disorders, heart disease and cancer. Chronic pain is often linked with depression. Who wouldn't be depressed in the face of unrelenting pain?

Inflammation is the underlying cause

Joint pain and back pain are most often caused by deterioration of the cartilage that cushion joints (including the spaces between the vertebrae, causing back pain), causing bone to rub against bone, resulting in inflammation and pain. This can be caused by an injury, but most often, it is the result of 40, 50, 60 years or even more of wear and tear on the joints.

While osteoarthritis (the wear and tear type of arthritis) is not an absolute as we age, the Centers for Disease Prevention and Control reports that 50% of us who are over 65 are diagnosed with osteoarthritis.

For most of us, our first remedy is to reach for aspirin, ibuprofen, or naproxen. That can be a fatal mistake. NSAIDs (non-steroidal anti-inflammatory drugs) like aspirin, ibuprofen, and naproxen plus a handful of prescription drugs like Celebrex, Anaprox, Feldene, and Voltaren can cause serious toxicity problems that require hospitalization for as many as 200,000 Americans each year and kill as many as 30,000 people. Yet 60 million of us use them regularly and doctors still happily prescribe them.

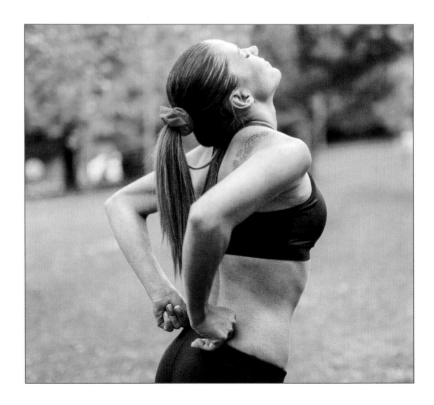

NSAIDs relieve inflammation by inhibiting the activity of an inflammation-causing enzyme called COX-2. That's all well and good, but they also inhibit a companion enzyme called COX-1, which protects the lining of the digestive tract and blood vessels. Therefore, without adequate COX-1 protection, you may have ulcers and leaking of the blood vessels.

Additionally, NSAIDs reduce kidney function, which can increase blood pressure and fluid retention and double or triple your risk for heart attack and stroke. That's a big price to pay for pain relief. There are safer ways to effectively reduce pain and inflammation.

NSAIDs are fine to treat acute inflammation occasionally, but long-term and regular use can be deadly.

Curcumin is the safe alternative

It shouldn't surprise you that curcumin and its formidable anti-inflammatory properties offer a powerful, yet safe, alternative to these dangerous NSAIDs. It does not affect healthy levels of COX-1 at all. In fact a study from our group published in *Cancer Letters* in 2001 showed that curcumin is a selective and specific blocker of COX-2 activity, and did not have any impact on COX-1 levels in colorectal cancer cells.

Curcumin works differently from NSAIDs in that curcumin modulates inflammatory pathways in the body without seriously impeding any one of them. The result is a reduction in inflammation shown in clinical studies to be every bit as good as, or even better, than these NSAIDs, all without the risks and negative effects!

Inflammation causes pain, so if you relieve inflammation, you relieve pain. Not only does curcumin relieve inflammation and pain, it can actually help rebuild worn cartilage, restoring joints to their youthful flexibility. Curcumin is also such a potent antioxidant that it can actually help repair the oxidative damage caused by inflammation.

Curcumin is no doubt a frontrunner and worthy of special recognition and status among healing plants. Medicines should heal, not hurt. They should promote life, not take it away. Many people seek natural remedies to alleviate pain, in part due to a belief that natural remedies are safer than most pharmaceuticals. But where do they look? Enter curcumin that can erase pain quickly and powerfully without negative effects.

The research is very impressive:

Reduce inflammation: Biological indicators of inflammation were reduced by as much as 99% with curcumin, offering almost complete relief for chronic pain sufferers and providing powerful promise for prevention and treatment of other diseases caused by inflammation.

Cartilage regeneration: Not only does curcumin help reduce the inflammation, it actually helps prevent the breakdown of cartilage (the cushion between joints), preventing arthritis from developing or worsening, as shown by Canadian researchers. At least one study shows that curcumin can help build new cartilage cells, reversing what was once thought to be an incurable degenerative disease.

Pain relief: An Italian study showed that people diagnosed with knee osteoarthritis were able to reduce their need for NSAIDs by 63% when they took curcumin. As a welcome side effect in this study, it was discovered that curcumin produced a 16-fold *reduction* in participants' blood levels of CRP, the protein that indicates high levels of inflammation, which also predicts a high risk for heart attack.

Rheumatoid arthritis (RA): My research found that curcumin works better than the most commonly prescribed NSAID treatment for rheumatoid arthritis. The results showed that curcumin outperformed diclofenac sodium (Voltaren) in reducing tenderness and swelling of joints in 45 participants who had active rheumatoid arthritis. It took just 500 mg of a high absorption curcumin blended with turmeric essential oils a day to equal the results we saw in people getting 50 mg of Voltaren—but all without side effects. In fact, 14% of the people in the drug group of this RA trial had to drop out due to severe side effects. How many people dropped out of the curcumin group? Zero. We also saw slightly more benefits in people who took a combination of the two, which shows us that there were no problems with combining curcumin with this type of prescription drug.

A landmark 2006 study from the University of Arizona takes the idea of inflammation a step further with the finding that curcumin might *prevent* rheumatoid arthritis, an autoimmune disease. Another study showed that curcumin was at least as effective as two commonly prescribed pain relievers for rheumatoid arthritis.

This adds up to substantial evidence that curcumin is a potent anti-inflammatory that addresses joint pain and works at least as well as—if not better than prescription drugs without the risk of side effects.

WHAT YOU NEED TO KNOW

- Conventional medicine most often treats back and joint pain with non-steroidal anti-inflammatories (NSAIDs), which can have life-threatening side effects. Curcumin provides equal or greater relief without side effects, instead conferring side "benefits."

- Curcumin can help regenerate cartilage tissue.

- Curcumin may prevent rheumatoid arthritis and people with the disease can get relief from curcumin without side effects.

CHAPTER 10

Obesity and Diabetes

Type 2 diabetes and its almost inextricable connection to being overweight and obese are the scourges of modern society. These terrible diseases and their side effects are direct results of a modern lifestyle heavy on processed foods, sugar and unhealthy types of fat. These diseases—yes, obesity is a disease—are already extracting a heavy price in terms of our national health, productivity, and quality of life.

This is a country where "food" (I say this in quotes intentionally) is more abundant than at any time in history. Empty calories from highly processed foods, junk foods and sugary soft drinks have made 17% of our children obese, creating a health crisis that will plague us for decades to come.

We also have chemicals and manipulated ingredients that have never before existed in our food chain, which worsens this problem.

Our lack of attention to healthy food choices is the disease of modern society. It's one we can and must change.

Obesity

Obesity has reached alarming proportions in the Western world. At least 69% of American adults are overweight, 35% of them are obese.

Being overweight, particularly with belly fat, is a well-documented cause of inflammation. Recent research has linked high-sugar, high-fat diets with changes in the immune cells and increased inflammation. As you know from the earlier chapters in this book, inflammation is an underlying cause of cancer and a number of other diseases, including diabetes.

At least one study calls curcumin an "anti-lipidemic," meaning it fights fat accumulation as well as inflammation and oxidative stress, all of which play important roles in obesity.

In fact, diabetes is intimately associated with obesity: 86% of all people diagnosed with Type 2 diabetes are overweight or obese.

Research published in the *British Journal of Nutrition* in 2011 confirmed that BCM-95™ curcumin reduces liver inflammation, neutralizing the risk for fatty liver disease associated with obesity.

Several studies show that curcumin can result in better blood sugar control and has been shown to cause a small, but significant decrease in body weight and body fat. Perhaps more importantly, curcumin also increases levels of a protein called adiponectin that is usually low in obese people. By raising adiponectin levels, normal weight can return. Curcumin also helps cut off the blood supply to excess fat cells, reducing their size and number.

In the simplest of terms, most of us need to get our weight under control for a number of reasons. Curcumin not only helps with weight control, it reduces the risk of diabetes even if you might be carrying a few extra pounds.

Obesity and diabetes are key factors for most cancers. If we can control these two conditions, we can effectively prevent cancer or manage it better.

Diabetes

Type 2 diabetes is the disease of the Western lifestyle. This disease, once known as adult-onset diabetes, was considered the province of the over-50 crowd. There were stereotypes of people with pot bellies, sitting in front of the TV, munching on potato chips chased with half a gallon of their favorite soft drink and a pint of Rocky Road. While this was likely true in some cases, it is a disservice to think that it is merely a disease of gluttony. Some people may have thought they had a healthy diet because of the emphasis in the last decades on low-fat, high-carb everything.

Now Type 2 diabetes is also the disease of teens raised on poor food choices, fast-food soy-enhanced, processed cheeseburgers, loads of refined carbs and gallons of sugary soda. It's now the disease of 20-somethings with high cholesterol,

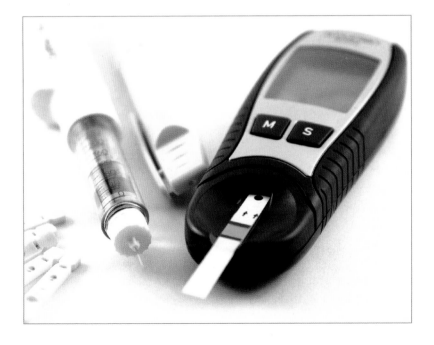

30-somethings with erectile dysfunction and 40-somethings with coronary bypasses and kidney failure.

Type 1 diabetes is usually diagnosed in children and is characterized by a malfunctioning pancreas that does not produce sufficient quantities of the body's own insulin to properly utilize the natural sugars in food.

Type 2 diabetes, on the other hand, is almost always a lifestyle disease. Scientifically, it is characterized by the body's inability to respond to the insulin produced by the pancreas. This is called insulin resistance.

The American Diabetes Association reports that more than 29.1 million Americans, or 9.3% of the U.S. population, have diabetes. Sadly, more than 8.3 million have no idea that they are suffering from this disease that has such far-reaching health consequences. Another 86 million are considered "pre-diabetic," meaning they have some blood sugar malfunction.

Worse yet, 25.9% of Americans over 65 have diabetes and 1.7 million new cases are diagnosed each year. It's the 7th leading cause of death in the U.S.

It's important to note that the vast majority of people with Type 2 diabetes are obese. Alarmingly, the number of people with diabetes in the U.S. has increased by 76% in the last 20 years on pace with the increase in obesity.

I'll repeat the figure I mentioned a few paragraphs back because it is so important: *86% of people diagnosed with Type 2 diabetes are overweight or obese.*

Living with blood glucose testing, dietary restrictions, and diabetes meds with a wide variety of side effects is only the tip of the diabetes iceberg.

Deadly complications

The complications of diabetes are daunting:

- Heart disease is reported as a cause of death in 68% of people with diabetes aged 65 and over.

- People with diabetes have a 2 to 4 times greater chance of dying of heart disease or stroke than those without the disease.

- High blood pressure is reported in 67% of those with diabetes.

- Diabetes is the leading cause of new cases of blindness in people aged 29–74.

- Kidney failure attributed to diabetes accounts for 44% of all new cases. In 2008, the latest year for which statistics are available, more than 202,000 people with end-stage kidney disease due to diabetes were living on dialysis or with a kidney transplant.

- Nerve damage is experienced by 60 to 70% of people with diabetes, often causing erectile dysfunction in men.

- Diabetes causes circulatory problems that led to 65,700 lower limb amputations in diabetics in 2008.

- Diabetes is listed as a contributing cause of death in more than 231,000 deaths.

Science now generally accepts that diabetes is an inflammatory condition, as is obesity. As you might well imagine, this is where curcumin comes into the picture.

Here's what research confirms curcumin can do:

Reduce glucose production in the liver: A Japanese study shows that curcumin has the ability to reduce the liver's natural production of the storage form of glucose, which in healthy people is balanced by the pancreas' production of insulin to keep glucose levels steady.

Keep glucose out of red blood cells: Scientists treated red blood cells to mimic diabetes, and then exposed them to curcumin for just 24 hours. The results: Curcumin normalized the cells in terms of sugar processing and prevented the formation of the fatty globules that clog arteries.

Prevent the development of diabetes: A Columbia University study showed that mice, with a predisposition toward diabetes and obesity, given daily doses of curcumin were less likely to develop impaired blood sugar, insulin resistance and full-blown diabetes than those that did not receive curcumin.

Lower blood sugar, increase insulin: Indian researchers found that curcumin contains a particularly powerful antioxidant that lowers blood sugar, increases insulin in the bloodstream (meaning existing insulin is being properly used) and protects against fatty deposits in the arteries indicative of heart disease.

Promote wound healing: Curcumin also helps in the process of wound healing, something that is especially important to people with diabetes, since their wound healing capabilities are often impaired, leading to infection and amputations.

Protect kidneys: It has also been found to protect the kidneys, which we know are vulnerable in people with diabetes, and to help prevent glaucoma and cataracts, common complications among people with diabetes.

Reverse diabetes: Probably one of the most exciting studies came from Egypt in 2008, when researchers discovered curcumin and a bone marrow transplant reversed diabetes in mice with the disease. Researchers theorized that the anti-inflammatory and antioxidant properties of curcumin enhanced the ability of the bone marrow transplant to regenerate insulin-producing cells. We can only hope to see human studies soon.

The evidence is abundantly clear: Curcumin has profound effects against one of the most deadly diseases of our time. Its pathways of action are widely varied and it is effective against a number of the complications of diabetes as well. While doctors are not yet ready to tell every person with diabetes to take curcumin, they are probably lagging behind the research curve. If I had diabetes, wild horses couldn't keep me away from my curcumin. I don't have diabetes, but curcumin is still a staple of my supplement regimen.

WHAT YOU NEED TO KNOW

◆ Obesity and Type 2 diabetes go hand in hand. Both are diseases caused by fat accumulation, inflammation and oxidative stress.

◆ Curcumin not only fights inflammation, as we have seen in many diseases, it also fights the accumulation of fat and oxidative stress—the perfect combination to combat both diseases.

◆ Curcumin helps regulate weight-regulating levels of adiponectin, regulates blood sugar and the production of insulin, reduces the storage form of glucose (glycogen) production in the liver, keeps glucose out of red blood cells, promotes wound healing, protects kidneys and can prevent the development of Type 2 diabetes and in some cases can reverse the disease.

CHAPTER 11

Heart Disease

Since heart disease is the #1 killer in the Western world, any nutrient that helps protect your heart and arteries and even helps reverse heart disease, should be most welcome.

Curcumin is that unique nutrient. Curcumin's heart protective effects become even more important when we add diabetes to the mix.

Heart disease is the most common complication of diabetes and the number of newly–diagnosed diabetics is increasing dramatically every year, with nearly 2 million new cases reported among U.S. adults in 2010. It killed 787,000 people in 2011, more than all forms of cancer combined.

Heart disease is also the #1 killer of women in the U.S., although only 1 in 5 women is aware of that grim fact.

Science has long known that heart disease is caused by inflammation, so curcumin's ability to combat inflammation is a major part of its effectiveness against heart disease in its many forms.

Keep arteries clear

Clogged arteries raise the risk of heart attack and stroke. Fatty deposits (called plaque) cause arteries to narrow, reduce blood flow, and make your heart work harder to move blood through the circulatory system and hardening the arteries. In time, this buildup can completely block an artery and cause a heart attack or stroke.

But what causes this process in the first place? Inflammation. As the arteries are irritated, nicked and stretched, they become inflamed. Then the inflammation causes further damage. The body detects the damage and sends Band-Aids to the site. These bandages are made of white blood cells, calcium and cholesterol. They are deposited on the injured site. The more places where bandages are placed, the narrower the blood vessel becomes. So cholesterol is not the cause of heart disease per se, but merely a result of the real culprit—inflammation.

It is generally protective of the heart to raise HDL cholesterol. Curcumin raises the levels of HDL or "good" cholesterol that helps move fats out of the cells, including the cells in the arteries. It also reduces the stickiness of blood cells, helping to prevent blood clots.

With curcumin, HDL cholesterol increases can happen fast: An Indian study showed that human volunteers who took 500 mg a day for just a week increased their good (HDL) cholesterol by 29%.

Other studies suggest that curcumin may actually bring

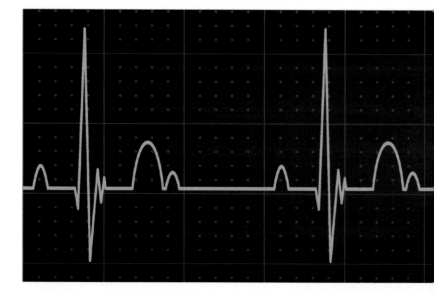

about epigenetic changes in the genes that signal the body to build up those fatty deposits in the arteries. Turning off those genes can help clear arteries.

Reduce homocysteine and CRP levels

Homocysteine is an amino acid naturally present in the human body. When homocysteine starts to build up in the bloodstream to higher than normal levels, it irritates the lining of the blood vessel. This increases the hardening and narrowing of the arteries, may cause blood clotting, raises your risk of heart disease and can be predictive of a heart attack, stroke and possibly Alzheimer's disease.

CRP (C-Reactive Protein) is one of the body's signals that inflammation is present. It is produced when inflammatory damage occurs. High levels of CRP may indicate that there is damage to the arterial walls. Damaged arterial walls trigger the atherosclerotic process (hardening of the arteries). Curcumin helps to relax those arterial wall cells, reduces the hardening of the arteries and allows the blood to flow more freely, dissolving clots, preventing and even reversing plaque buildup.

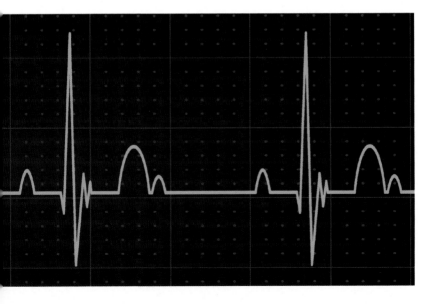

Reverse heart failure

Congestive heart failure occurs when the heart muscles can no longer pump enough blood to the rest of the body. It is usually a slow process that gets worse over time. The heart muscles lose their ability to pump oxygen-rich blood throughout the body, causing fluid buildup in the lungs, liver, gastrointestinal tract, arms and legs. This lack of oxygen damages vital organs, eventually causing death.

Curcumin prevents the thickening of the heart muscle leading to the creation of scar tissue in the heart muscle and helps failing hearts return to their normal pumping capacity, according to breakthrough 2016 Indian animal research. Scientists at the University of Calcutta found that curcumin caused epigenetic changes that allowed low-dose highly absorbable forms of the rhizome to work effectively to reverse heart failure.

Other animal research confirms that curcumin stops heart function from deteriorating, especially in people with diabetes who are particularly prone to heart failure.

Heart failure is sometimes the result of a heart attack, it can also be caused by diabetes, thyroid disease, alcohol, drug abuse and HIV/AIDS. Heart failure can also be caused by moving to a high altitude (elevation over 10,000 feet) or constant heavy exercise.

Prevent stroke and stop stroke damage

Strokes have two major causes. The most common is a blood clot that travels to the brain and the second is a ruptured blood vessel in the brain. As we learned earlier in this chapter, the buildup of cholesterol, elevated homocysteine and CRP levels, and even congestive heart failure, are risk factors for stroke as well as heart attack. Since stroke is a cardiovascular disease, a stroke is a "brain attack," if you will, similar to a heart attack.

We already know that curcumin has powerful preventive and healing properties for all of these conditions.

Strokes almost inevitably damage brain cells. But exciting new research shows that curcumin, given intravenously, can minimize brain damage while a stroke is in progress because it can cross the blood-brain barrier, protecting the mechanisms that help regenerate brain cells if it is administered in an emergency room within three hours of a stroke. Unfortunately, intravenous curcumin is not standard in hospitals in the United States, but these studies show the tremendous promise of curcumin.

Curcumin's ability to protect your heart, brain and cardiovascular system is very impressive. Consider the drugs commonly used to treat the heart conditions discussed in this chapter. The statin drugs alone (Lipitor, Crestor and their cousins) carry with them huge health risks from side effects, including causing death from sudden heart failure. Blaming cholesterol for heart disease is like blaming a bandage for your skinned knee. Therefore, these drugs are not as effective at preventing heart attacks as you might think.

It only makes sense to use nutrients like curcumin that are highly effective as well as having an excellent safety profile.

Curcumin is natural and safe. Only rarely do people taking curcumin get mild stomach upset at very large dosages of 10 grams per day or more. And with today's innovations in improving curcumin's absorption, using 10 grams a day is no longer necessary.

What's more, even the highest quality products are very affordable. Who could ask for more?

WHAT YOU NEED TO KNOW

- Curcumin's anti-inflammatory effects should make it an important part of any strategy to fight heart disease.

- Curcumin raises HDL "good" cholesterol, helping move fats out of arteries and reduces the stickiness of blood cells, preventing abnormal blood clots.

- Curcumin reduces markers for inflammatory CRP and homocysteine, reducin the risk of heart disease.

- Curcumin has been shown to reverse congestive heart failure and reduce the risk of stroke and brain damage from strokes.

CHAPTER 12

Digestive Disorders

Time after time, curcumin has proven its value in treating a wide variety of digestive disorders, largely because of its anti-inflammatory effects.

Digestive disorders range from mild indigestion to life controlling conditions like irritable bowel syndrome and celiac disease to life threatening diseases like ulcerative colitis and colorectal cancer.

My research has generally focused around colorectal cancers and frequently it spills over into other aspects of digestive disorders. Of course, colorectal cancer is a digestive disorder, but I think I've adequately addressed all of the properties of curcumin for that specific type of cancer in earlier chapters.

Each year, 62 million Americans are diagnosed with some form of digestive disorder.

Irritable bowel syndrome, a complex and unpredictable set of painful problems ranging from diarrhea to constipation and cramping, bloating and pain, goes largely undiagnosed, with an estimated 75% of sufferers not getting medical treatment at all.

Colorectal cancer kills about 150,000 people every year and ulcerative colitis, celiac and Crohn's diseases make life miserable for 140,000 Americans.

Liver disease is included in this category because of the liver's key role in the digestive process.

Curcumin to the rescue

Because inflammation is a major factor in all digestive disorders, curcumin is predictably very effective in helping prevent, treat, and heal many digestive problems.

Herbalists consider curcumin to be a digestive and a bitter, which means it helps ease digestion and aids liver function.

It also stimulates bile production in the liver and improves the ability to digest fats.

Here's a listing of various digestive disorders and how curcumin can help:

Irritable bowel syndrome: Irritable bowel syndrome is an unpleasant cluster of problems that fluctuate between diarrhea and constipation with abdominal cramps, bloating, and gas in the mix. A study from the Medical College of Wisconsin helps us understand better the anti-inflammatory capabilities of cur-

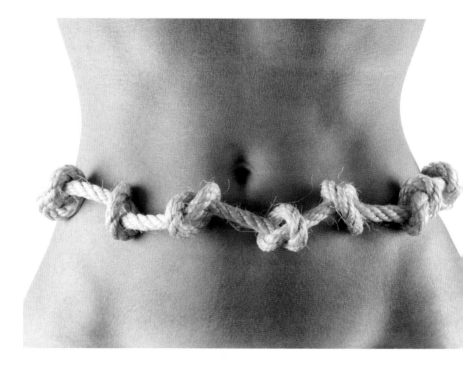

cumin, which stops the growth of additional blood vessels to feed the inflamed area in the digestive tract. This is a form of angiogenesis, which we've covered in earlier chapters on its role in cancer.

Crohn's disease: Researchers at M.D. Anderson Cancer Center in Houston recommend we "get back to our roots" and take advantage of the anti-inflammatory effects of curcumin for many diseases, including Crohn's, an inflammatory disease usually affecting the large and small intestines. Crohn's and ulcerative colitis are sometimes called inflammatory bowel disease.

Ulcerative colitis: This Japanese study, which involved human subjects, a rarity in curcumin research to this point, suggests curcumin supplements are a safe way of preventing recurrences of the disease and reducing the side effects, which include severe bleeding, ruptured colon, dehydration and liver disease.

Colon cancer: We've already examined curcumin's anticancer properties in detail, but it's worth mentioning it again here. A landmark study from the American Health Foundation shows that curcumin interferes with the process by which malignant colon tumors develop, stopping them before they become dangerous.

Familial adenomatous polyposis: In a study published in the journal *Clinical Gastroenterology and Hepatology*, five patients with an inherited form of precancerous polyps in the lower bowel known as familial adenomatous polyposis (FAP) were treated with regular doses of curcumin and quercetin (another powerful antioxidant found in onions and garlic) over an average of six months. The average number of polyps dropped 60.4%, and the average size dropped by 50.9%.

Liver damage: An interesting Finnish animal study involved feeding rats a diet that simulated high alcohol consumption.

Animals given curcumin at the same time had none of the signs of liver damage normally associated with alcoholism. Researchers theorize that curcumin blocks a molecule called NFkB, which is responsible for inflammation and tissue death. Another study showed that animals with 70% of their livers removed were able to start to grow new liver tissue in as little as 24 hours with the help of curcumin.

Other digestive problems: The research on curcumin and gastrointestinal diseases is pretty impressive, but there is more. Extensive research also confirms its value in treating gastric and peptic ulcers as well as gall stones and gall bladder inflammation.

Once again, curcumin proves its considerable value in fighting inflammation with remarkable results in treating, preventing and stopping the progress of a variety of digestive disorders. Its effects on treating and preventing liver disease, a potentially fatal affliction, are even more remarkable.

WHAT YOU NEED TO KNOW

- Curcumin's anti-inflammatory effects help prevent and treat a wide variety of digestive disorders.

- For people with irritable bowel syndrome, curcumin can provide relief by reducing the blood supply to the inflamed area of the colon.

- Curcumin has also been shown to stop the growth of precancerous polyps in the lower bowel known as familial adenomatous polyposis.

- Animal studies show that curcumin protects the liver from damage from excess alcohol use as well as helping grow new liver tissue.

CHAPTER 13

Message to Healthcare Practitioners

Most authors are very protective of their work and prohibit copying and distributing book contents unless they are sold or pay a fee.

This section of the book is very different. This information is so important that I want to see it distributed far and wide. At least as far as this chapter goes, I am unconcerned about copyright.

I also know that doctors and other healthcare practitioners are very busy. They are very unlikely to read an entire book, even though, like this book, it may contain some information that could save the lives or help improve the quality of life of their patients. I understand that doctors are frequently skeptical about natural formulations and, if they haven't conducted their own research investigations on a subject, they are inclined to steer their patients away from them, even though these formulations might be life saving.

So I've created this very short chapter, a synopsis of the most important elements of this book. I encourage you to copy it freely. Give it to your doctor or other healthcare practitioner and encourage him or her to spend 10 minutes reading and digesting these short pages.

Dear Doctor,

Your patient has given you a copy of this chapter with my bless-ings and permission. My publisher and I have given it to the pub-lic domain so that the vital information it contains on curcumin's value in prevention and treatment of a wide range of cancers can be broadly circulated.

I have spent more than 20 years researching the chemo-preventive and treatment properties of curcumin. I've published more than 200 studies on various aspects of health and cancer, including the health benefits of complementary and alternative medicine. I am convinced that curcumin can offer broad benefits to prevent, treat, and perhaps even cure cancer with virtually no side effects.

Of course, I am not the only researcher investigating cur-cumin's benefits. More than 8,200 studies have been published on curcumin's medical benefits, most of them within the last 15 years. A search of the electronic database of the National Insti-tutes of Health (NIH) called PubMed (available at pubmed.gov) on curcumin and cancer returns 3,132 results as of this writing. Many of these studies are well constructed and highlight the scientific merit for this natural medicine.

In brief, this is what we've learned about curcumin and its effects on cancer cells and the genes that govern them:

Anti-inflammatory

Curcumin is one of the most potent plant-based, naturally occur-ring, anti-inflammatory substances known to science. It has virtu-ally no side effects or toxicity, even when taken in large amounts. As a side note: Cancer rates in my native India are very low, which may largely be due to the universal dietary consumption of cur-cumin (as turmeric) and other spices with medicinal properties. Curcumin:

- Inhibits the COX-2 and NF-Kappa B inflammatory pathways, preventing chronic inflammation.

◆ It scrubs away the free radical oxygen molecules inhibiting the production of inflammatory arachidonic acid.

◆ It controls cytokine production.

◆ It slows or stops production of other enzymes, including protein kinase.

EPIGENETICS

This relatively new field of science investigates gene expression in cancer and confirms that lifestyle and environmental changes can restore healthier and more balanced genetic expression, preventing and treating cancer. Curcumin:

◆ Helps control the expression of important genes that cause cancer to spread.

◆ Reactivates quiescent tumor-suppressing genes and down-cycles tumor-promoting genes.

◆ Controls the expression of many miRNAs that control the growth and behavior of cancers-causing genes.

APOPTOSIS, ANGIOGENESIS, METASTASIS

Programmed cell death, prevention of angiogenesis to nurture cancer cells, and prevention of metastasis are essential to all forms of cancer treatment today. Curcumin:

◆ Induces apoptosis through a variety of pathways.

◆ Inhibits angiogenesis signaling pathways more effectively than angiogenesis inhibitors.

◆ Inhibits EGFR and VEGF pathways that control cancer spread.

◆ Anti-metastatic natural medicine.

◆ Blocks inflammatory pathways, including metastasis in advanced cancers, including pancreatic, liver and colorectal.

CANCER STEM CELLS

Cancer stem cells are largely responsible for recurrence months or even years after treatment. Curcumin:

◆ Disrupts signaling pathways, prevents communication with other cancer cells and prevents recurrence.

◆ Increases the ability of chemotherapy to kill cancer stem cells.

CHEMO-RESISTANCE

In my experience, almost every cancer patient develops chemo-resistance at some point in the treatment cycle. Curcumin:

◆ Helps overcome chemo-resistance, enhancing the effectiveness of chemotherapy drugs.

◆ Neutralizes cancer cellular survival mechanisms.

CHEMO-SENSITIZER

On the other side of the same coin, curcumin has been shown to "open" cancer cells to chemotherapy treatments. Curcumin:

◆ Sensitizes cancer cells and cancer stem cells to a variety of chemotherapy drugs.

◆ Improves effectiveness of commonly used chemotherapy agents, including 5-FU.

◆ Enhances the effectiveness of several drugs used to treat advanced colon cancers, including irinotecan, FOLFOX, gemcitabine, celecoxib and paclitaxel for breast cancer.

◆ Improves effectiveness of chemotherapy drugs in a variety of cancers: breast, colon, pancreas, gastric, liver, blood, lung, prostate, bladder, cervix, ovary, head and neck. This includes advanced cancers that are considered inoperable.

◆ Activates miRNAs to overcome chemo-resistant cancer stem cells.

◆ Protects healthy organs, especially liver, kidney, heart and oral mucosa from toxic effects of chemotherapy and radiation.

◆ Improves quality of life and increases survival time.

INTEGRATIVE THERAPY

Curcumin works synergistically in conjunction with many other natural substances. Curcumin:

- Enhances the effects of chemotherapy and protects surrounding tissue from damage caused by radiation and chemo drugs.

- Enhanced effectiveness when used in conjunction with a variety of other natural substances, including boswellia, Omega-3 fatty acids, vitamin D, resveratrol and green tea.

Research from Harvard and Massachusetts General Hospital confirms that the effectiveness of a cocktail including curcumin could have "potent anti-tumor" effects, enhancing the effects of all types of therapies while reducing the toxicity of chemotherapy and radiation treatments. Ingredients in the cocktail: curcumin, oleic acid (found in olive oil), silibinin (from milk thistle), EGCG (from green tea), kaempferol (found in many foods, including onions and green tea), melatonin, enterolactone (plant lignans found in a wide variety of foods including seeds, whole grains and legumes), withaferin A (an Ayurvedic herb) and resveratrol (from red grapes).

Curcumin has been studied and found effective for the following types of cancer:

- Colorectal
- Breast
- Pancreatic
- Liver
- Lung
- Melanoma
- Bone
- Multiple myeloma
- Prostate
- Head and neck cancers
- Chronic myeloid leukemia
- Brain (glioblastoma)
- Gall bladder
- Lymphoma
- And many other types of cancer

OTHER INFLAMMATORY DISEASES

Curcumin has been validated as an effective agent against a wide variety of other diseases, at least in part due to its anti-inflammatory properties.

Among them, in addition to cancer, other diseases include:

◆ Obesity

◆ Heart Disease

◆ Diabetes

◆ Arthritis and chronic pain

◆ Depression

◆ Dementia and Alzheimer's disease

◆ Digestive disorders including Crohn's disease, ulcerative colitis, irritable bowel syndrome, familial adenomatous polyposis, alcohol-induced liver damage

ALL CURCUMIN IS NOT CREATED EQUAL

It's important to note here the difference between turmeric and curcumin and the difference between various types of curcumin.

Turmeric is a culinary spice with definite health benefits if used in large quantities on a daily basis. Curcumin, if extracted properly from the turmeric rhizome, is highly bioavailable and highly therapeutic. In simple terms, turmeric is the spice, curcumin is the natural medicine, present in this spice.

Furthermore, I am often asked if all curcumin extracts are the same. The answer is simply, "no." It's important to pay attention to the quality of the extract, including whether it has higher absorption and does not contain any harsh, toxic chemicals used during its extraction from the turmeric rhizome. The BCM-95™ formulation, which I've used exclusively in my research, is extracted using non-toxic methods and has been well researched as the most bioavailable of all curcumin extractions on the market today. It is both absorbable and therapeutic and is prepared based upon traditional principles of Ayurvedic medicine.

I strongly urge you not only to encourage your patients to use curcumin, but to find a formulation that will have the most therapeutic effects for treating cancer and a broad range of other inflammatory diseases.

CONCLUSION

In my mind, curcumin is one of the most exciting substances we have found to prevent, treat and potentially even cure cancer. Not only does it affect more than 700 genes, curcumin also affects more than 100 different cellular pathways. Multiple studies have shown it to be safe in the treatment of all cancers with no toxicity even at high doses.

This brief overview may have whetted your appetite to learn more. If so, I encourage you to get a copy of the entire book and investigate some of the research for yourself.

I hope you will add curcumin to your arsenal for your patients, particularly for those with cancer.

Thank you for bearing with me and hearing this message.

Ajay Goel, Ph.D.

CHAPTER 14

Take-Home Message

I'm not a superlative kind of guy. I'm a scientist and I admit I'm kind of a geeky one, as you might expect. I spend endless hours in my lab searching out every detail in my research, looking at it from every angle and actively seeking flaws.

That's why I am extremely excited about the potential of curcumin to bring about healing in ways that medical science has not yet fathomed.

When I started writing this book, I thought I'd slowly ease you into all of these ideas about how curcumin attacks cancer:

- Inflammation
- Epigenetics
- Apoptosis
- Angiogenesis
- Metastasis

- Cancer stem cells
- Chemo-resistance
- Chemo-enhancement
- Protection for tissue damage from chemo-therapy and radiation

My editor warned me that if I threw out all of these frankly amazing benefits of curcumin in the first chapter, I'd be branded a snake oil salesman, readers would doubt my credibility and they'd be unlikely to read the subsequent chapters that document the scientific proof of the power of curcumin against cancer.

Now that you've read the explanations and the science, when you add them all up, there is no doubt at all that curcumin works like no other substance we know to attack cancer from many angles without serious side effects. It is the antithesis to modern medicine's arsenal of toxic drugs to treat cancer, many of which harm as much as they help.

Curcumin works like no other substance known to science, pharmaceutical or natural, to attack cancer and overcome it.

So now we need to take a look at the best ways to incorporate curcumin in your preventive regimen and, if you've been diagnosed with cancer, we'll look at formulations that target cancer in a variety of ways.

Bioavailability vs. bioactivity

Many studies emphasize curcumin's low *bioavailability*. That means that the human body can't easily access the nutrients and health benefits it offers. In simple terms, we're talking about absorption into the blood through the digestive tract.

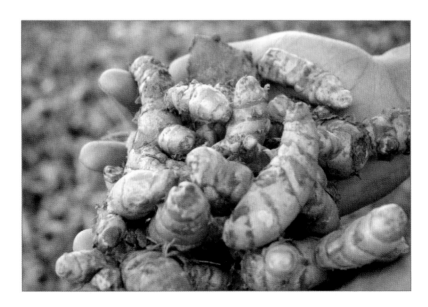

Despite the controversy that curcumin is poorly absorbed because low levels of it are detectable in blood, thousands of published studies confirm curcumin's effectiveness in treating and preventing a broad range of diseases, including cancer. This suggests curcumin doesn't work like an aspirin—you can't swallow it with a glass of water and it takes care of the problem. That means it *must* work in another way. What we know for sure is that it *does* work!

Low blood levels of curcumin are not at all a deal breaker. Let's explore a little painless biochemistry first.

There are four basic reasons why curcumin doesn't show up in large amounts in the bloodstream:

1. Low water solubility

2. Poor absorption through the digestive tract

3. Metabolic conversion of the curcumin after consuming it, making it hard to detect in blood

4. Binding of curcumin to cellular proteins in various body tissues, resulting in less curcumin circulating in the bloodstream

Low water solubility

Low water solubility is not a problem for digestive cancers, particularly colorectal cancer, since curcumin is absorbed along the digestive tract in exactly the way any food is absorbed. Water is not necessary for this action.

Curcumin is fat soluble. When it is taken by mouth, curcumin is detectable in the brain, which may in part explain its effectiveness in preventing and treating brain diseases.

Other new research suggests that the parent curcumin molecule may not be the most important part here. It's a case of the child becoming more powerful than the parent. Research shows us that when curcumin is processed by the liver, it is broken down into many components, each of which has its own benefits. Some of those metabolites of curcumin have their own anti-tumor and anti-inflammatory effects, adding to their effectiveness against cancer and other diseases.

It's also possible that many of curcumin's components have already been used by the body (metabolized) by the time blood is tested to determine if they are still present. In addition, some of them are known to be water soluble and they will show up in blood tests, but they are no longer recognizable as curcumin.

Best bioavailability

I'm not going to recommend specific products here, but there is one formulation of curcumin that I have used in my research, called BCM-95® that makes it much more bioavailable than ordinary curcumin supplements, which are only 50 to 60% absorbed by weight. This means the curcumin's absorption can be seen in blood tests.

The BCM-95® extraction process blends curcumin with essential oils from turmeric based on the centuries-old Ayurveda system, so the product is all natural. It has been shown to have 7 to 10 times higher bioavailability and research shows it is retained longer in the circulatory system than standard curcumin. There are curcumin products that claim higher bioavailability, but their fatty coating is synthetic. Additionally, it is very important to note that turmeric essential oil contains turmerones, which are themselves anticancer and have been shown to boost the activity of curcumin.

One study shows that BCM-95® has a double peak action. It shows up in the bloodstream of human subjects within an hour and drops for a short period of time, then rises again 4.5 hours later and remains detectable in the blood after eight hours. That means not only is it absorbed, it remains in the system much longer than any other curcumin supplement, which typically dissipate within a little more than two hours.

The BCM-95® formulation is clearly superior, because it is easily absorbed and contains compounds (turmerones) that boost curcumin's effectiveness. I have used it in all of my research because several well-designed studies confirm that BCM-95® curcumin provides measurable health benefits. It is also one of the most clinically studied, enhanced absorption curcumin products available in the U.S. under the TERRY NATURALLY brand name CuraMed® from EUROPHARMA

Conclusion

Anyone who has had cancer knows that doctors are extremely reluctant to proclaim that a patient is "cured." Yet that is the word every patient and every family member wants to hear.

Yes, we know that doctors will say a patient is in remission or even long-term remission after 5 or 10 years have passed cancer-free. However, many doctors and patients feel the shadow of cancer may again rise up. They are correct—sometimes it does.

Yet, I am boldly saying today that we are approaching the time when curcumin will enable us to actually prevent cancer and possibly cure patients, even some with late-stage cancers. More research is needed, but curcumin's promise in dealing with cancer has already been repeatedly validated.

Right now, we can say with confidence that curcumin enables people with almost every kind of cancer to live longer, sometimes much longer, than was originally projected when they were diagnosed.

Cancer treatment is a very personal choice.

I encourage people with cancer to discuss this book with their practitioners and decide, after weighing all the evidence, if curcumin is right for them.

Whether you decide to pursue active mainstream treatment or decide to avoid these treatments, curcumin can play an important role in your health.

And those who choose curcumin in combination with conventional treatments that usually include chemotherapy and radiation can rest assured that they are enhancing the effectiveness of those therapies while protecting healthy tissues from the side effects of those treatments that can ravage the body.

As a side note: If you have been diagnosed with cancer and your doctor is uncertain whether curcumin might be harmful or interact negatively with conventional treatment, please copy Chapter 13 and encourage your medical practitioners to read it. It is short and succinct and should dispel any worries.

Yet most important for those who are healthy and wish to remain healthy (who doesn't?), curcumin offers effective prevention, not only against almost all types of cancer, but also against other debilitating diseases, including diabetes, heart disease, obesity, Alzheimer's, depression, digestive disorders, arthritis and joint pain.

Curcumin can prevent you from tipping the scales toward these diseases due to epigenetic, environmental and lifestyle causes.

If you know you are at risk for any of these diseases, start taking a high quality curcumin formulation immediately.

If you have been diagnosed with any disease I've mentioned here, it is my strong belief that you would benefit from a high quality curcumin supplement.

If you have been diagnosed and treated for cancer, I strongly urge you to take curcumin and continue taking it every day for the rest of your life to prevent cancer stem cells from bringing about a recurrence.

As I mentioned earlier in this book, I am of Indian descent and I know I have a family tendency toward diabetes. I watch my diet carefully, especially when I travel, and I take curcumin every single day, without fail. I will continue to do so for the rest of my life.

I hope you will do so as well.

References

Chapter 1: Why We're Losing the War on Cancer

Cancer statistics:

1950 Mortality Data—CDC/NCHS, NVSS, Mortality Revised. 2002 Mortality Data: US Mortality Public Use Data Tape, 2002, NCHS, Centers for Disease Control and Prevention, 2004

http://www.csicop.org/si/show/war_on_cancer_a_progress_report_for _skeptics/

http://www.cancerresearchuk.org/cancer-info/cancerstats/world/ incidence/#By

Simmons, D. Epigenetic Influence and Disease. *Nature Education* 2008; 1(1):6.

Chapter 2: Cancer is an Inflammatory Disease

Jurenka, JS. Anti-inflammatory Properties of Curcumin, a Major Constituent of *Curcuma longa:* A Review of Preclinical and Clinical Research. *Alternative Medicine Review* 2009 Jun:14(2):141–53.

Lim J, Iyer L, et al. Diet-Induced Obesity, Adipose Inflammation, and Metabolic Dysfunction Correlating with Par2 Expression Are Attenuated by PAR2 Antagonism. *The FASEB Journal* 2013;27(12):4757.

Gregor MF, Hotamisligil GS. Inflammatory Mechanisms in Obesity. *Annual Review of Immunology* 2011;29:415–45. Review.

Lumeng CN, Saltiel AR. Inflammatory Kinks Between Obesity and Metabolic Disease. *Journal of Clinical Investigations* 2011;121(6):2111–2117.

Howe LR, Subbaramaiah K. Molecular Pathways: Adipose Inflammation as a Mediator of Obesity-Associated Cancer. *Clinical Cancer Research.* 2013 Nov 15;19(22):6074–83.

Hursting SD, DiGiovanni J, et al. Obesity, Energy Balance and Cancer: New Opportunities for Prevention. *Cancer Prevention Research.* 2012; 5:1260–72.

Chapter 3: Curcumin: Getting Back to Our Roots

Barres R et al. Acute Exercise Remodels Promoter Methylation in Human Skeletal Muscle. *Cellular Metabolism* 2012;15:405–11.

Goel A, Kunnumakkara AB et al. Curcumin as "Curecumin": From Kitchen to Clinic. *Biochemistry Pharmacology* 2008 Feb 15;75(4):787–809. Epub 2007 Aug 19.

Jurenka JS. Anti-inflammatory Properties of Curcumin, a Major Constituent of *Curcuma longa:* a Review of Preclinical and Clinical Research. *Alternative Medicine Review* 2009 Jun;14(2):141–53.

Chapter 4: Epigenetics: Awakening Sleeping Genes

Toden S, Goel A. The Importance of Diets and Epigenetics in Cancer Prevention: A Hope and Promise for the Future? *Alternative Therapies in Health and Medicine* 2014;20(suppl 2):6–11.

Barres R et al. Acute Exercise Remodels Promoter Methylation in Human Skeletal Muscle. *Cellular Metabolism* 2012:15;405–11.

Reuter S, Goel A et al. Epigenetic Changes Induced by Curcumin and Other Natural Compounds. *Genes and Nutrition* 2011 May;6(2):93–108. doi: 10.1007/s12263-011-0222-1.

Wang Z, et al. Broad targeting of angiogenesis for cancer prevention and therapy. *Seminars in Cancer Biology* (2015) Dec;35 Suppl:S224–43. doi: 10.1016/j.semcancer.2015.01.001. Epub 2015 Jan 16.

Shanmugam MK, Rane G et al. The Multifaceted Role of Curcumin in Cancer Prevention and Treatment. *Molecules* 2015 Feb 5;20(2):2728–69. doi: 10.3390/molecules20022728.

Chapter 5: How Cancer Starts, Stays and Spreads

Bhandarkar SS, Arbiser IL. Curcumin as an Inhibitor of Angiogenesis. *Advances in Experimental Medicine and Biology.* 2007;595:185–95.

Bandyopadhyay D. Farmer to Pharmacist: Curcumin as an Anti-Invasive and Antimetastatic Agent for the Treatment of Cancer. *Frontiers in Chemistry* 2014 Dec 23;2:113. doi: 10.3389/fchem.2014.00113. eCollection 2014.

Koff J, Ramachandiran S et al. A Time to Kill: Targeting Apoptosis in Cancer. *International Journal of Molecular Sciences* 2015;16:2942–2955. doi:10.3390/ijms16022942.

Chapter 6: Stop Cancer from Returning

Goel, A and Aggarwal, BB. Curcumin, the Golden Spice From Indian Saffron, Is a Chemosensitizer and Radiosensitizer for Tumors and Chemoprotector and Radioprotector for Normal Organs. *Nutrition and Cancer* 2010;62(7);919–930.

Kim YS, Farrar W et al. Cancer Stem Cells: Potential Target for Bioactive Food Components. *Journal of Nutritional Biochemistry* 2012;23:691–698.

Norris L, Karmokar A et al. The Role of Cancer Stem Cells in the Anti-Carcinogenicity of Curcumin. *Molecular Nutrition and Food Research* 2013; 57;163–167.. Doi 10.1002/mnfr.201300120.

Saha S, Adhikary A et al. Death by Design: Where Curcumin Sensitizes Drug-resistant Tumours. *Anticancer Research* 2013;32:2567–2584.

Li Y, Zhang T. Targeting Cancer Stem Cells by Curcumin and Clinical Applications. *Cancer Letters* 2014;346:197–205.

Kakarala M, Brenner D et al. Targeting Breast Stem Cells with the Cancer Preventive Compounds Curcumin and Piperine. *Breast Cancer Research and Treatment* 2010 Aug;122(3):777–85. doi: 10.1007/s10549-009-0612-x. Epub 2009 Nov 7.

Kim YS, Farrar W et al Cancer Stem Cells: Potential Target for Bioactive Food Components. *Nutritional Biochemistry.* 2012 Jul;23(7):691–8. doi: 10.1016/j.jnutbio.2012.03.002.

Kakarala M, Brenner DE et al. Targeting Breast Cancer Stem Cells with the Cancer Preventive Compounds Curcumin and Piperine. *Breast Cancer Research and Treatment.* 2010 Aug;122(3):777–85. doi: 10.1007/s10549-009-0612-x. Epub 2009 Nov 7.

Shakibaei M, Goel A et al. Curcumin Enhances the Effect of Chemotherapy Against Colorectal Cancer Cells by Inhibition of MF-kB and Src Protein Kinase Signalling Pathways. *PLoS One.* 2013;8(2):e57218. doi: 10.1371/journal.pone.0057218. Epub 2013 Feb 22.

Chapter 7: Curcumin as an Integrative Therapy

Toden S, Goel A et al. Curcumin Mediates Chemosensitization to 5-fluoro-uracil through miRNA-induced Suppression of Epithelial-tomesenchymal Colorectal Cancer. *Nutrition and Cancer,* 2010:62:7;919–930.

Goel A, Aggarwal BB. Curcumin, the Golden Spice from Indian Saffron, Is a Chemosensitizer and Radiosensitizer for Tumors and Chemoprotector for Normal Organs. *Carcinogenesis* 2015 Mar;36(3):355–67. doi: 10.1093/carcin/bgv006.

Toden S, Goel A et al . Novel Evidence for Curcumin and Boswellic Acid Induced Chemoprevention through Regulation of miR-34a and miR-27a in Colorectal Cancer. *Cancer Prevention and Research* 2015 Feb 23. pii: canprevres.0354.

Frenkel M, Abrams D et al. Integrating Dietary Supplements Into Cancer Care. *Integrative Cancer Therapies* 2013;12(5):369–384.

Toden S, Goel A et al. Novel Evidence for Curcumin and Boswellic Acid-Inducted Chemoprevention through Regulation of miR-34A and miR-271 in Colorectal Cancer. *Cancer Prevention Research* 2015 May;8(5): 431–43. doi: 10.1158/1940-6207.CAPR-14-0354. Epub 2015 Feb 23.

Sethi S, Li Y et al. Regulating miRNA by natural agents as a new strategy for cancer treatment. *Current Drug Targets* 2013 Sep;14(10):1167–74.

Siddiqui RA, Harvey KA et al. Characterization of Synergistic Anticancer Effects of Docosahexaenoic Acid and Curcumin on DMBA-induced Mammary Tumorigenesis in Mice. *Biomed Central Cancer* 2013 Sep 13;13:418. doi: 10.1186/1471-2407-13-418.

Wang Z, Dabrosin C et al. Broad Targeting of Angiogenesis for Cancer Prevention and Therapy. *Seminars in Cancer Biology* 2015 Jan 16. pii: S1044-579X(15)00002-4. doi: 10.1016/j.semcancer.2015.01.001.

Kunnumakkara AB, Guha S et al. Curcumin Potentiates Anti-tumor Activity of Gemcitabine in an Orthotopic Model of Pancreatic Cancer through Suppression of Proliferation, Angiogenesis, and Inhibition of Nuclear factor-kappaB-regulated Gene Products. *Cancer Research* 2007 Apr 15;67(8): 3853–61.

Shakibaei N, Goel A et al. Curcumin Potentiates Anti-tumor Activity of 5-fluorouracil in a 3D Alginate Tumor Microenvironment of Colorectal Cancer. *Biomed Central Cancer* 2015 Apr 10;15:250. doi: 10.1186/ s12885-015-1291-0.

Patel VB, Misra S, et al. Colorectal Cancer: Chemopreventive Role of Curcumin and Resveratrol. *Nutrition and Cancer* 2010 Oct;62(7):958–67.

Xu G, Ren G et al. Combination of Curcumin and Green Tea Catechins Prevents Dimethylhydrazine-induced Colon Carcinogenesis. *Food and Chemical Toxicology* 2010 Jan;48(1):390–5.

Bartik L, Whitfield GK et al. Curcumin: A Novel Nutritionally Derived Ligand of the Vitamin D Receptor with Implications for Colon Cancer Chemoprevention. *Journal of Nutritional Biochemistry* 2010 Jan;48(1):390–5. doi: 10.1016/j.fct.2009.10.027.

Chapter 8: Depression, Alzheimer's and Dementia

Sanmukhani J, Goel A et al. Efficacy and Safety of Curcumin in Major Depressive Disorder: A Randomized Controlled Trial. *Phytotherapy Research* 2014 Apr;28(4):579–85. doi: 10.1002/ptr.5025.

Lopresti AL, Maes M et al. Curcumin and Major Depression: A Randomised, Double-blind, Placebo-controlled Trial Investigating the Potential of Peripheral Biomarkers to Predict Treatment Response and Antidepressant Mechanisms of Change. *European Neuropharmacology* 2015 Jan;25(1):38–50. doi: 10.1016/j.euroneuro.2014.11.015.

Choudhary KM, Mishra A et al. Ameliorative Effect of Curcumin on Seizure Severity, Depression Like Behavior, Learning and Memory Deficit in Post-pentylenetetrazole-kindled Mice. *European Journal of Pharmacology* 2013 Mar 15;704(1–3):33–40. doi: 10.1016/j.ejphar.2013.02.012.

Feng HL, Fan H et al. Neuroprotective Effect of Curcumin to A[Beta] of Double Transgenic Mice with Alzheimer's Disease. *Zhonggup Zhong Yao Za Zhi* 2014 Oct;39(19):3846–9. (Article in Chinese.)

Ringman JM, Frautschy SA, et al. A Potential Rose of the Curry Spice Curcumin in Alzheimer's Disease. *Current Alzheimer's Research.* 2005 Apr; 2(2): 131–136.

Yang F, Lim GP et al. Curcumin Inhibits Formation of Amyloid Beta Oligomers and Fibrils, Binds Plaques and Reduces Amyloid in Vivo. *Journal of Biological Chemistry.* 2005 Feb 18;280(7):5892–901. Epub 2004 Dec 7.

Michra S, Palanivelu K. The Effect of Curcumin (Turmeric) on Alzheimer's Disease: An Overview. *Annals of Indian Academy of Neurology* Jan;11(1): 13–9. Doi: 10.4103/0972-2327.40220.

Chapter 9: Arthritis and Joint Pain

Chandran B, Goel A. A Randomized, Pilot Study to Assess the Efficacy and Safety of Curcumin in Patients with Active Rheumatoid Arthritis. *Phytotherapy Research* 2012 Nov;26(11):1719–25. doi: 10.1002/ptr.4639.

Goel A, Boland CR. Specific Inhibition of Cyclooxygenase-2 (COX-2) Expression by Dietary Curcumin in HT-29 Human Colon Cancer Cells. *Cancer Letters.* 2001 Oct. 30;172(2):111–8.

Antony B, Kizhakedath R et al. Clinical Evaluation of an Herbal product (Rhulief™) in the Management of Knee Osteoarthritis. Abstract 316. *Osteoarthritis Cartilage.* 2011;19(S1):S145–S146.

Belcaro G, Dugall M et al. Meriva®+Glucosamine Versus Condroitin+ Glucosamine in Patients with Knee Osteoarthritis: An Observational

Study. *European Review for Medical and Pharmacological Sciences* 2014; 18(24):3959–63.

Nonose N, Pereira JA et al. Oral Administration of Curcumin (Curcuma longa) Can Attenuate the Neutrophil Inflammatory Response in Zymosan-Induced Arthritis in Rats. *Acta cirúrgica brasileira* 2014 Nov; 29(11):727–34.

Rao TS, Basu N et al. Anti-Inflammatory Activity of Curcumin Analogues. *Indian Journal of Medical Research.* 1982 Apr;75:574–8.

Funk JL, Frye JB et al. Efficacy and Mechanism of Action of Turmeric Supplements in the Treatment of Experimental Arthritis. *Arthritis and Rheumatology.* 2006 Nov;54(11):3452–64.

Joe B, Nagaraju A et al. Mass-Spectrometric Identification of T-kininogen I/thiostatin as an Acute-phase Inflammatory Protein Suppressed by Curcumin and Capsaicin. *PLoS One* 2014 Oct 9;9(10):e107565. doi: 10.1371/journal.pone.0107565. eCollection 2014.

Chapter 10: Obesity and Diabetes

Lerav V, Freuchet B et al. Effect of Citrus Polyphenol- and Curcumin-Supplemented Diet on Inflammatory State in Obese Cats. *British Journal of Nutrition* 2011 Oct;106 Suppl 1:S198–201. doi: 10.1017/S0007114511002492.

Uysal KT, Wiesbrock SM et al. Protection from Obesity-induced Insulin Resistance in Mice Lacking TNF-alpha Function. *Nature* 1997; 389:610–14.

Na LX, Yan BL et al. Curcuminoids Target Decreasing Serum Adipocyte-fatty Acid Binding Protein Levels in Their Glucose-Lowering Effect in Patients with Type 2 Diabetes. *Biomedical and Environmental Sciences.* 2014 Nov;27(11):902–6. doi: 10.3967/bes2014.127.

Qian Y, Zhong P et al. A Newly Designed Curcumin Analog Y20 Mitigates Cardiac Injury via Anti-Inflammatory and Antioxidant Actions in Obese Rats. *PLoS One* 2015 Mar 18;10(3):e0120215. doi: 10.1371/journal.pone .0120215. eCollection 2015.

Ghorbani Z, Hekmatdoost A et al. Anti-hyperglycemic and Insulin Sensitizer Effects of Turmeric and its Principle Constituent Curcumin. *International Journal of Endocrinology and Metabolism* 2014 Oct 1;12(4):e18081. doi: 10.5812/ijem.18081. eCollection 2014.

Rashid K, Sil PC. Curcumin Enhances Recovery of Pancreatic Islets from Cellular Stress Induced Inflammation and Apoptosis in Diabetic Rats. *Toxicology and Applied Pharmacology* 2015 Feb 1;282(3):297–310. doi: 10.1016/j.taap.2014.12.003.

Cruz-Correa M, Shoskes DA et al. Combination Treatment with Curcumin and Quercetin of Adenomas in Familial Adenomatous Polyposis. *Clinical Gastroenterology and Hepatology.* 2006 Aug;4(8):1035–8. Epub 2006 Jun 6.

Marquardt JU, Gomez-Quiroz L et al. Curcumin Effectively Inhibits Oncogenic NF-Kappa-B Signaling and Restrains Stemness Features in Liver Cancer. *Journal of Hepatology.* 2015 Sep;63(3):661–9. doi: 10.1016/j.jhep.2015.04.018. Epub 2015 May 1.

Chapter 11: Heart Disease

Soni KB, Kuttan R. Effect of Oral Curcumin Administration on Serum Peroxides and Cholesterol Levels in Human Volunteers. *Indian Journal of Physiology and Pharmacology.* 1992 Oct;36(4):273–5.

Ramaswami G, Chair H et al. Curcumin Blocks Homocysteine-induced Endothelial Dysfunction in Porcine Coronary Arteries. *Journal of Vascular Surgery* 2004 Dec;40(6):1216–22.

Shar BH, Nawaz Z. Inhibitory Effect of Curcumin, a Food Spice from Turmeric, on Platelet-activating Factor- and Arachidonic Acid-mediated Platelet Aggregation Through Inhibition of Thromboxane Formation and Ca2+ signaling. *Biochemical Pharmacology* 1999 Oct 1;58(7):11 67–72.

Fujiwara H1, Hosokawa M. Curcumin Inhibits Glucose Production in Isolated Mice Hepatocytes. *Diabetes Research and Clinical Practice.* 2008 May;80(2):185–91. doi: 10.1016/j.diabres.2007.12.004. Epub 2008 Jan 24.

Yang FW, Liu C et al. Effects of Three Kinds of Curcuminoids on Anti-Oxidative System and Membrane Deformation of Human Peripheral Blood Erythrocytes in High Glucose Levels. *Cellular Physiology and Biochemistry.* 2015;35(2):789–802. doi: 10.1159/000369738. Epub 2015 Jan 30.

Maithilikarpagaselvi N, Sridhar MG. Curcumin Prevents Inflammatory Response, Oxidative Stress and Insulin Resistance in High Fructose Fed ale Wistar Rats: Potential Role of Serine Kinases. *Chemico-Biological Interactions.* 2015 Dec 20;244:187–194. doi: 10.1016/j.cbi.2015.12.012. [Epub ahead of print]

Ray A, Rana SA et al. Improved Bioavailability of Targeted Curcumin Delivery Efficiently Regressed Cardiac Hypertrophy by Modulating Apoptotic Load within Cardiac Microenvironment. Toxicology and Applied Pharmacology 2016 Jan 1;290:54–65.

Zhao J, Zhao Y et al. Neuroprotective Effect of Curcumin on Transient Focal Cerebral Ischemia in Rats. *Brain Research* 2008 Sep 10;1229:224–32.

Tummalapalli M, Berthet M, Composite Wound Dressings of Pectin and Gelatin with Aloe Vera and Curcumin as Bioactive Agents. *International Journal of Biological Macromolecules.* 2016 Jan;82:104–13. doi: 10.1016/j.ijbiomac.2015.10.087. Epub 2015 Nov 1.

Najafi H, Changizi Ashtiyani S. Therapeutic Effects of Curcumin on the Functional Disturbances and Oxidative Stress Induced by Renal Ischemia/Reperfusion in Rats. *Avicenna Journal of Phytomedicine*. 2015 Nov-Dec;5(6):576–86.

El-Azab MF, Attia FM. Novel Role of Curcumin Combined with Bone Marrow Transplantation in Reversing Experimental Diabetes: Effects on Pancreatic Islet Regeneration, Oxidative Stress and Inflammatory Cytokines. *European Journal of Pharmacology* 2011;658:41–48.

Chapter 12: Digestive Disorders

Gupta SC, Patchva S et al. Therapeutic Roles of Curcumin: Lessons Learned from Clinical Trials. *American Association of Pharmaceutical Scientists Journal* 2013 Jan;15(1):195–218. doi: 10.1208/s12248-012-9432-8.

Bundy R, et al. Turmeric Extract May Improve Irritable Bowel Syndrome Symptomology on Otherwise Healthy Adults: A Pilot Study. *Journal of Alternative and Complementary Medicine* 2004 Dec;10(6):1015–8.

Kumar A, Purwar B et al. Effects of Curcumin on the Intestinal Motility of Albino Rats. *Indian Journal of Physiology and Pharmacology* 2010 Jul-Sep;54(3):284–8.

Hanai H, Iida T et al. Curcumin Maintenance Therapy for Ulcerative Colitis: Randomized, Multicenter, Double-Blind, Placebo-Controlled Trial. *Clinical Gastroenterology and Hepatology*. 2006 Dec;4(12):1502–6. Epub 2006 Nov 13.

Kawamori T, Lubet R, et al. Chemopreventive Effect of Curcumin, a Naturally Occurring Anti-Inflammatory Agent, During the Promotion/Progression Stages of Colon Cancer. *Cancer Research* 1999 Feb 1;59(3):597–601.

Chapter 13: Message to Healthcare Practitioners

Wang Z, Dabrosin C et al. Broad Targeting of Angiogenesis for Cancer Prevention and Therapy. *Seminars in Cancer Biology*. 2015 Dec;35 Suppl: S224–43. doi: 10.1016/j.semcancer.2015.01.001. Epub 2015 Jan 16.

Chapter 14: Take Home Message

Shusuke T, Goel A. Invited Editorial: The Holy Grail of Curcumin and its Efficacy in Various Diseases: Is Bioavailability Truly a Big Concern? (unpublished).

Antony B, Benny M, et al. A Controlled Randomized Comparative Human Oral Bioavailability of "Biocurcumax™ (BCM-95® CG)—A Novel Bioenhanced Preparation of Curcuminoids. *Indian Journal of Pharmacological Sciences* 2008 Jul–Aug;70(4):445–9.

Index

About the Author

Ajay Goel, Ph.D., is a professor and director of the Center for Gastrointestinal Research and Center for Epigenetics, Cancer Prevention and Cancer Genomics at the Baylor Research Institute, Baylor University Medical Center in Dallas, TX.

He has spent more than 20 years researching cancer and has been the lead author or contributor to more than 200 peer-reviewed scientific articles published in leading international journals and several book chapters. He is currently researching basic and translational aspects of gastrointestinal cancer prevention through a variety of approaches, including the use of complementary and integrative botanical products. Two of the primary botanicals he is investigating are curcumin (from turmeric) and boswellia.

Dr. Goel is a member of the American Association for Cancer Research and the American Gastroenterology Association and serves on the editorial boards of more than a dozen journals including *Gastroenterology, Clinical Cancer Research, PLoS One, Epigenomics, Future Oncology, Scientific Reports* and *Alternative Therapies in Health and Medicine.* He also performs peer-reviewing activities for more than 100 scientific journals, as well as serves on various grant-funding committees of the National Institutes of Health and various international organizations.